Spinal Cord Blood Supply:
In-Depth Look

Georgia

TABLE OF CONTENTS

<u>THE BLOOD SUPPLY OF THE HUMAN SPINAL CORD AT BIRTH</u>

INTRODUCTION

The pattern of the blood vessels of the central nervous system as displayed in the fully developed human foetus and in the human neonate, is also the adult pattern. Streeter (1918), observed: "It is possible to subdivide the development of the blood vessels of the brain into 5 successive periods, each showing special adaptations to their changing environmental conditions ..... under the fifth period we would include the late histological changes in the walls of the vessels that convert them into the adult arteries, veins and the various types of sinuses."

For the purposes of this study, it has been assumed that the vessels of the spinal cord are to be seen in their optimal state in the new born and that a detailed record may serve as an anatomic baseline for the study of the adolescent, the adult and the senile patterns, in health and in disease. It has also been assumed that Streeter's observation in respect of the blood vessels of the brain, is valid when applied to the vessels of the remaining major portions of the central nervous system. The main stimulus for the study has been the lack of certainty in regard to the role of the arterial supply of the spinal cord, in spinal surgery - in particular, in the anterior approaches used in the management of scoliosis and of infective lesions such as tuberculosis.

Suh and Alexander (1939) commented, "most of what has been written in the past 40 years about the circulation of the human spinal cord ..... is either inaccurate or incomplete." While this comment is no longer necessarily justified, it is a fact that a review of the literature including many of the most recent publications, reveals a lack of unanimity which is disconcerting to the clinician and the practising surgeon.

Techniques of study have varied and have been as diversified as the reports which have resulted from their application. The variability of techniques and of reports is a measure of the complexity of the subject, and an indication also of the fact that without the advantages of a near-perfect injection technique, and the use of the binocular surgical microscope, it may be necessary to make assumptions and to bridge gaps while gathering data. Such assumptions are likely to prove faulty on closer inspection, and to be attributable to the abundant presence of greater and lesser vessels which criss-cross and overlap each other until the examiner is confused, and until a situation arises in which he is unable "to see the wood for the trees".

The complexity of the study is simplified when it is appreciated that the paired segmental vessels which are found at every inter-vertebral level, are for the supply of the surrounding structures, and that arterial feeder vessels occur only at scattered and variable levels in different individuals. The segmental arteries give off small branches even before arriving at the entrance to the inter-vertebral foramina, but it is at this situation that they break up and divide into their numerous branches for the supply of extra- and intra-vertebral structures.

THE SEGMENTAL ARTERIES

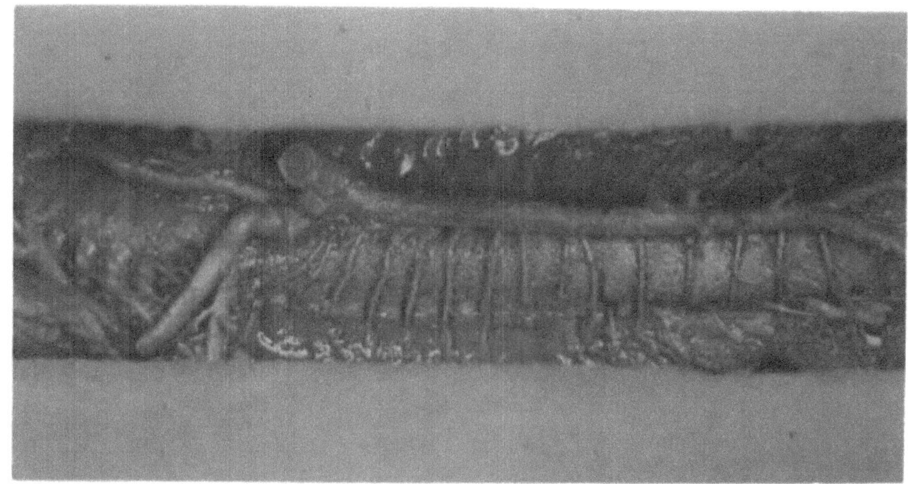

Fig. 1.   Cadaver 3212. A pair of arteries is found at every segmental level.
In the thoracic and the lumbar regions they arise from the back of the
Aorta, while in the cervical and the sacral regions, the source of their
origin is less regular. (x$\frac{1}{2}$).

The thoracic segmental arteries are commonly referred to as the intercostal arteries, noth-
withstanding the fact that the intercostal vessels are the terminal branches of the segmental
arteries. In order to avoid misunderstanding in the matter of terminology, and for the purposes of this dissertation, the terms "Aortic Segmental Artery" will be applied to these vessels in the thoracic and the lumbar areas, and the levels of their occurrence will be indicated,
thus: Aortic Segmental Artery, Thoracic 4, or in abbreviated form thus: A.S.A., T.4, or
A.S.A., L.2.

The segmental arteries proceed to the inter-vertebral foramina at their respect-levels, and
supply nutrient vessels to the vertebral bodies "en route".

They divide into their major branches at the foramina, which may be described as the "segmental distribution points".

THE SEGMENTAL ARTERIES

THE DISTRIBUTION POINT for the segmental arteries is at the inter-vertebral foramina, where they divide into a number of branches for the supply of the neighbouring extra- and intra-dural structures.

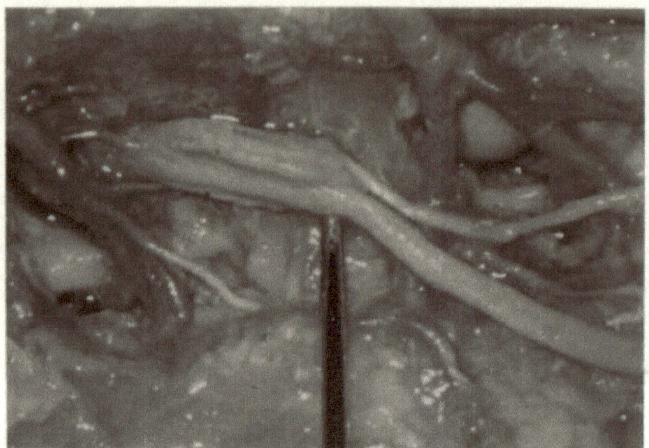

Fig. 2.   The "Distribution Point" of the segmental arteries is at the inter-vertebral foramen, where branches for the supply of intra- and extra-dural structures arise. The 12th Thoracic Nerve on the right side is seen emerging from the canal. (x25).

There are the anterior branches which are for the supply of the extra-spinal structures, and the posterior branches which supply the intra-spinal structures and the posterior skeletal apparatus.

The so-called "radicular arteries" or "spinal arteries" for the reinforcement of the anterior median and the postero-lateral arterial trunks of the spinal cord do not occur at all segmental levels; on the contrary, they are to be found at occasional levels only, and for the purpose of this dissertation will be referred to as the "feeder arteries".

The segmental arteries of the cervical and the lumbar regions arise variously from a number of sources. (Fig. 3, overleaf). In the neck they arise from the costo-cervical and the thyro-cervical trunks, and also from the vertebral arteries from within the bony canal in which they are housed in the neck. The external carotid contributes a number of segmental vessels too, in the cephalic portion of the neck. Branches from the ascending pharyngeal artery were observed, in 5 out of 6 specimens in which they were sought, and although they contributed to the blood supply of the extra-spinal structures and were also observed to form arterio-arterial anastomoses with branches of the ascending cervical and the vertebral arteries, they made no contribution in the form of feeder vessels to the spinal cord.

THE SEGMENTAL VERTEBRAL ARTERIES OF THE CERVICAL REGION

CEPHALIC ASPECT

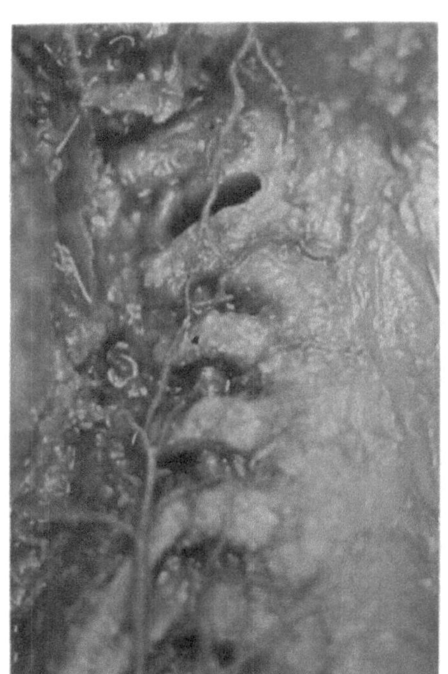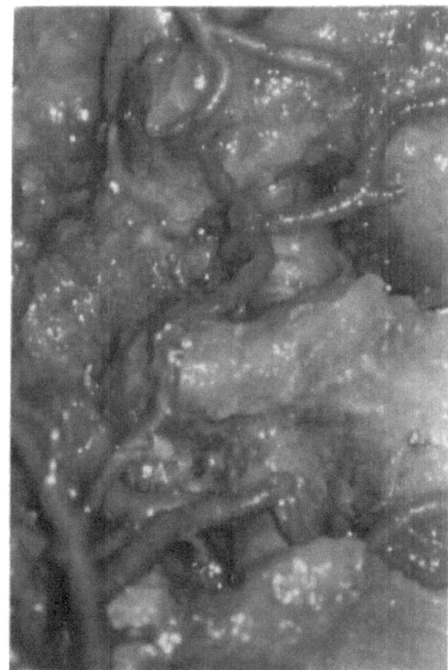

CAUDAL ASPECT

Fig. 3a.   The vertebral artery and the foramina transversaria on the right side from C.1 to C.6 levels. Multiple segmental arteries arise from the vertebral and the ascending cervical arteries, which also anastomose with each other and with a descending branch of the ascending pharyngeal artery. The longus colli muscle has been removed. (x10).

Fig. 3b.   Detail from fig. 3a, at C.2/3 and C.3/4 levels. The arterio-arterial anastomoses are well displayed. (x25).

THE SEGMENTAL VERTEBRAL ARTERIES OF THE SACRAL REGION

In the sacral and lumbo-sacral areas, there is involvement in the origin of segmental arteries of a number of vessels in varying degree. The source vessels include the aortic segmental artery, L.4, the ilio-lumbar artery, the middle sacral artery and the lateral sacral artery or arteries. The latter are of particular significance and were found to contribute feeder vessels in 7 of the 21 specimens in the series.

The segmental arteries at the various levels constitute an intimate part of the study of the feeder arteries of the spinal cord, and the important role which they play in the co-ordinated vascular supply of the spinal cord and surrounding structures can be fully appreciated only when the dissections are carried out with the spinal cord 'in situ'.

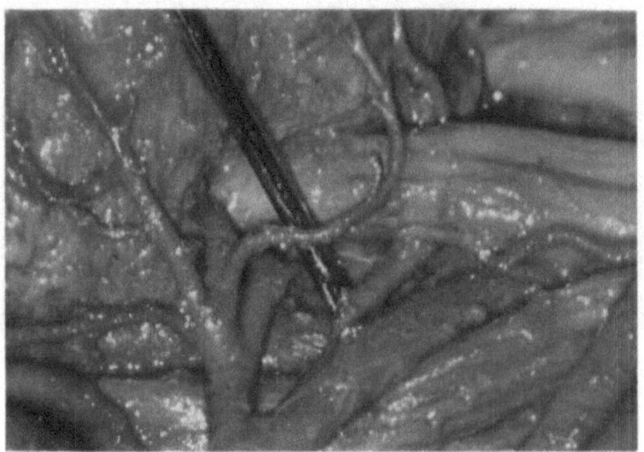

Fig. 4.   The first sacral nerve root on the right side is seen emerging from the foramen, which gives passage to segmental branches of the lateral sacral artery. An arterio-arterial anastomoses connects the first to the second lateral sacral artery. (x25).

THE ANTERIOR MEDIAN ARTERIAL TRUNK OF THE SPINAL CORD

The arterial supply of the spinal cord is derived from a single anterior arterial trunk which for the most part is placed on the median sulcus, and from a pair of postero-lateral arterial trunks which weave a tortuous course in close relationship to the posterior rootlets of the segmental nerves, from the upper cervical level down to the conus. When viewed from behind, the postero-lateral trunks are in large measure covered by the nerve rootlets, to the extent that their continuity has been disputed.

Terminology in respect of the anterior and the posterior channels is inclined to be confusing, and to leave doubts in the mind of the student when referred to simply as the "spinal arteries". For the purposes of this dissertation, the terms "Anterior Median Arterial Trunk" and "Postero-lateral arterial trunk" will be used throughout. The collateral arteries of supply of the three arterial trunks, commonly referred to as "radicular arteries", will be termed "arterial feeders", and the term "radicular artery" will be confined to those vessels which terminate in the nerve root and sheath.

PLATE I, in which the detailed findings in 3 cadavers are represented in the form of diagrams, will be followed on alternate pages by Plates II - VII, each of which records the anterior median arterial trunk and collaterals in 3 cadavers, and by Plate X in which the findings in 3 posterior dissections are accurately charted.

COMMENT ON PLATE I (see Plate overleaf).

Cadaver 3444. At the proximal extremity of the median trunk there are communications with the left and right vertebral arteries. The trunk is duplicated over a short distance, and diminishes in size, proximo-distally. It would seem reasonable to infer that the direction of flow is also in a proximo-distal direction. The presence of a large arterial feeder vessel in the cervical region, of two feeders of average size in the thoracic region, and of a larger median arterial trunk at the lumbar enlargement, is typical. The perforating sulcal arteries are prominent in the lumbar region.

Cadaver 3436. The median trunk is discontinuous at C.2 level. This is an unusual variation which was observed in one specimen only. Perforating sulcal arteries are prominent in the cervical and lumbar regions. The artery of Adamkiewicz is on the <u>right</u> side at T.11 level.

Cadaver 3447. At the proximal level, the median trunk communicates with the vertebral artery on the left side. An unusually large number of arterial feeders is present in the cervical region, and also at lumbar level. By contrast, the median arterial trunk for the thoracic cord is of average size only, having a diameter of 200 micro-millimeters. The artery of Adamkiewicz arises from aortic segmental artery, "A.S., L-3", on the left side.

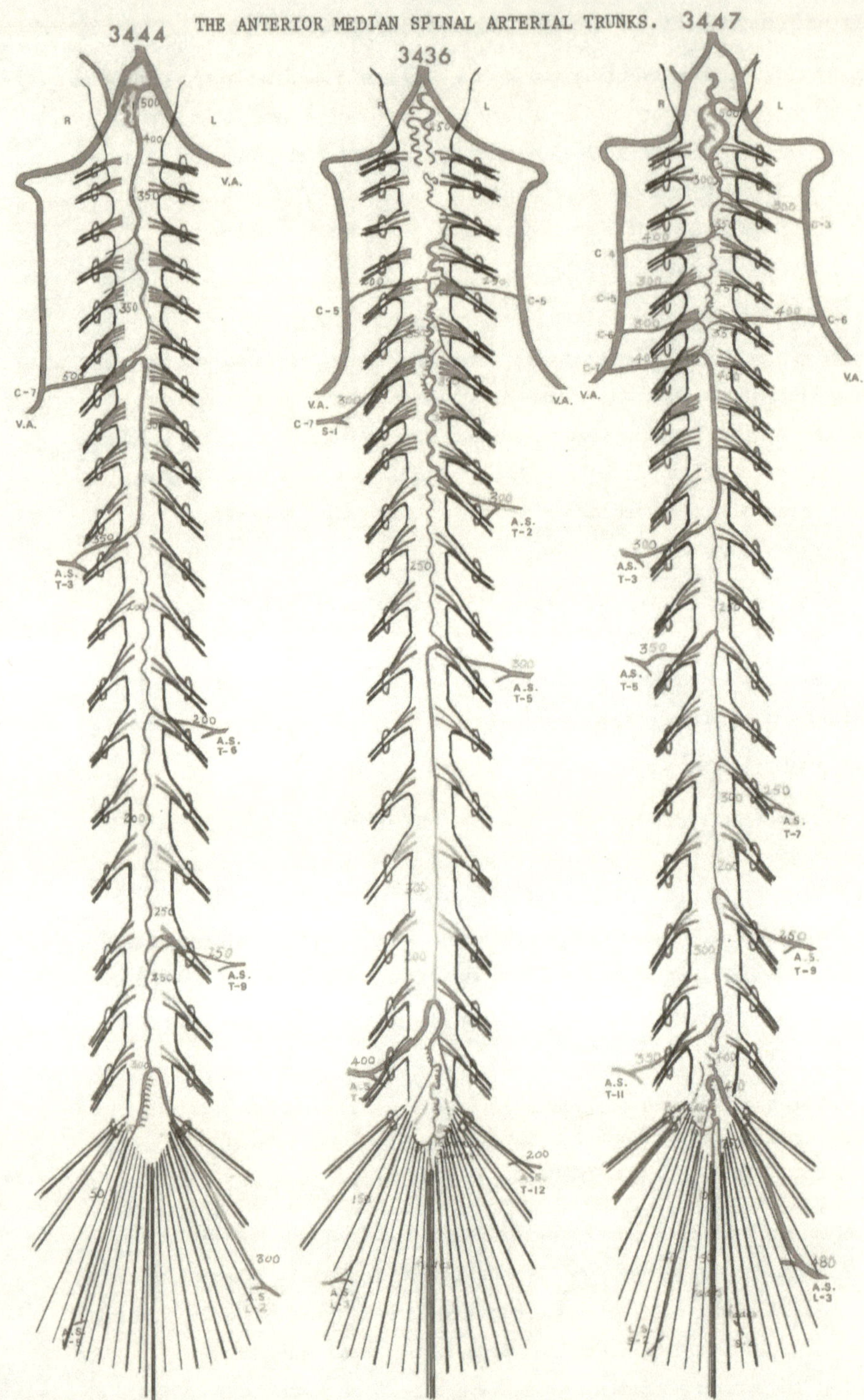

THE ANTERIOR MEDIAN SPINAL ARTERIAL TRUNKS.
3444
3436
3447
R
L
V.A.
C-5
C-7
V.A.
A.S.
T-3
A.S.
T-6
A.S.
T-9
C-5
C-7
S-1
V.A.
A.S.
T-2
A.S.
T-5
A.S.
T-12
C-4
C-5
C-6
C-7
C-3
C-6
V.A.
A.S.
T-3
A.S.
T-5
A.S.
T-7
A.S.
T-9
A.S.
T-11
A.S.
L-3
V.A. Vertebral Artery
A.C. Ascending Cervical Artery
D.C. Deep Cervical Artery
S.I. Superior Intercostal Artery
A.S. Aortic Segmental Artery (levels indicated)
I.L. ILIO—Lumbar Artery
L.S. Lateral Sacral Artery
The approximate size of the main arterial trunk and of each
feeder vessel is indicated, in terms of micro—millimeters
PLATE 1

THE ANTERIOR MEDIAN ARTERIAL TRUNK OF THE SPINAL CORD (continued)

COMMENT ON PLATE II

Cadaver 3288. The communications from the vertebral arteries to the median trunk at the proximal extremity form parallel trunks in the upper cervical region before uniting to form the median trunk. The ascending cervical artery contributes arterial feeders to the cervical cord on the right side, and on the left side there are 4 thoracic arterial feeders, including the artery of Adamkiewicz at T. 8 level.

A large posterior communicating artery is observed at the level of the conus medullaris, passing from the anterior median arterial trunk to the postero-lateral arterial trunk on the left side.

Cadaver 3292. At the proximal extremity, the communications between the anterior median trunk and the two vertebral arteries display an unusual configuration, and one may speculate about the direction of blood-flow. In the thoracic region the calibre of the median trunk is of average size, and in the lumbar region, there is a "pulled-up" appearance of the arterial feeder, typical for that region. It is attributed to the growth in a proximal direction of the spinal cord, which is tethered distally by the filum terminale. Well-developed posterior communicating branches are present at the conus, and the perforating sulcal arteries are prominent. There is no vessel to which the term "Adamkiewicz's artery" may be applied.

Cadaver 3301. At the proximal extremity, communications between the median arterial trunk and the vertebral artery are on the left side only. The small number of arterial feeder vessels is in strong contrast with the large number seen in the adjoining diagram, yet the concentration of enlarged channels is again in the cervical and the lumbar regions, and there is a thoracic channel which is of good average dimension.

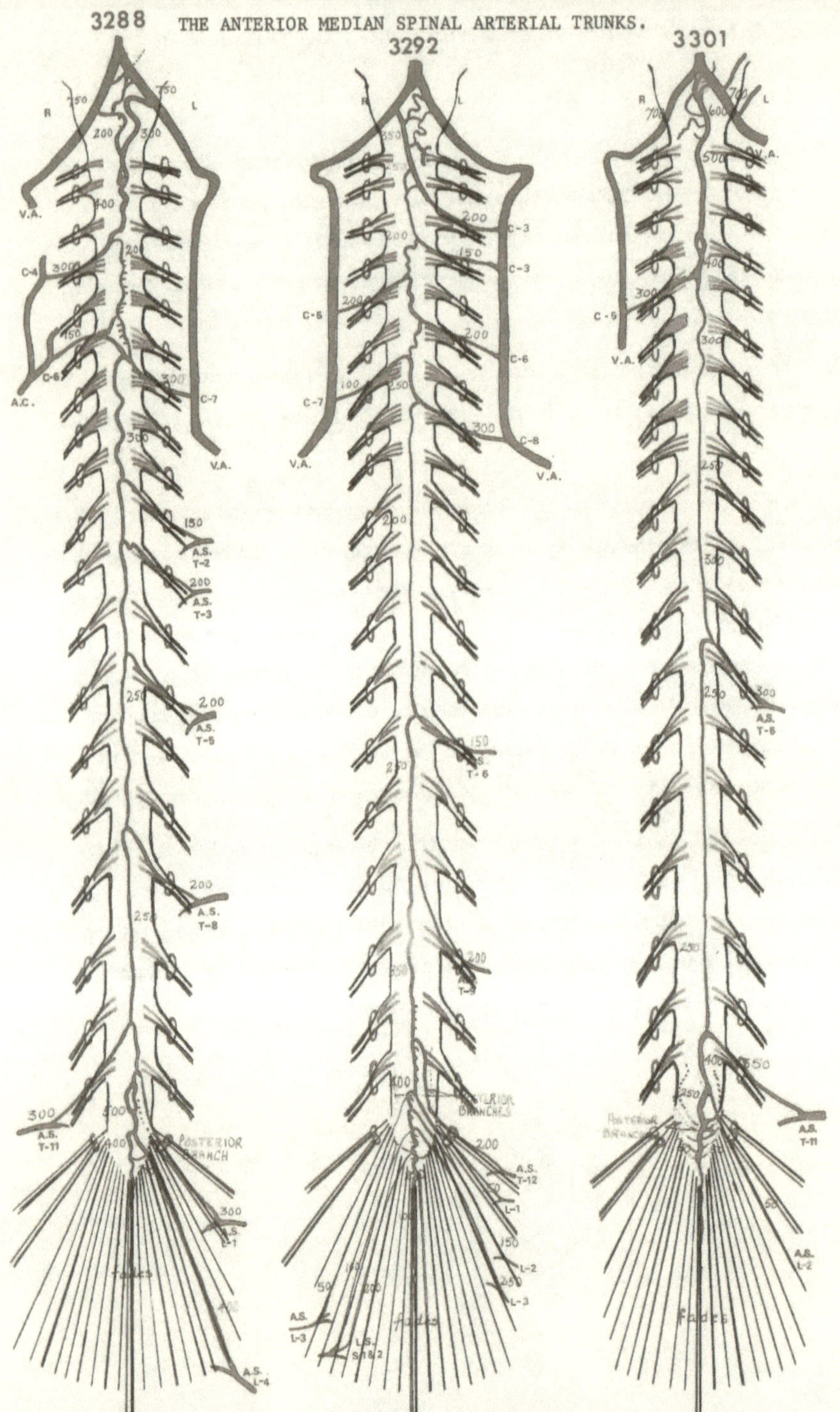

V.A. Vertebral Artery
A.C. Ascending Cervical Artery
D.C. Deep Cervical Artery
S.I. Superior Intercostal Artery

A.S. Aortic Segmental Artery (levels indicated)
I.L. ILIO—Lumbar Artery
L.S. Lateral Sacral Artery

The approximate size of the main arterial trunk and of each
feeder vessel is indicated, in terms of micro-millimeters

PLATE 2

THE ANTERIOR MEDIAN ARTERIAL TRUNK OF THE SPINAL CORD (continued)

The sequence of display of the dissections in the series is the sequence in which the dissections were carried out, and has not been arranged to illustrate a point. From each specimen, additional facts and interesting figures may be gleaned. Already, the great variability of pattern and the universal consistency of principle will be apparent: There is an abundance of arterial supply where the demand is greatest, namely, at the cervical and the lumbar enlargements of the cord. There is a less abundant vascularity in the upper and mid-thoracic regions where no neural enlargements are to be found. There appears to be an elasticity in the choice of the direction of flow of the blood volume at certain regions, notably at the proximal and the distal extremities.

COMMENT ON PLATE III:

Cadaver 3323. In the cervical region, the median arterial trunk diminishes in size as it proceeds in a cephalic direction, and the concept of the division of the arterial system of the spinal cord into three functional areas, namely, the area of the cervical enlargement, that of the less complicated upper thoracic region, and the lumbar enlargement, is supported by reference to the pattern displayed in this diagram.

The Y-shaped junctions between the collateral feeders and the median arterial trunk in the thoracic and the cervical regions, in contra-distinction to the inverted U-shape in the lumbar area, are well demonstrated in this and in the accompanying two diagrams.

Cadaver 3184. At the proximal extremity, the size of the main arterial channel at different levels would seem to suggest a flow of blood in a cephalic direction. Unusual features of this specimen are an arterial feeder at C.8 level, and a particularly large arterial feeder at T.5.

The left-sided preponderance of arterial feeders is well illustrated. The artery of Adamkiewicz is at T.9 level on the left side, and is larger than average.

Cadaver 3208. There are 17 arterial feeders, the largest number in the series. (see also figs. 5-9 on pages 32-35).

The principle of a copious blood supply in the region of the cervical and lumbar enlargements is upheld, while in the region of the thoracic cord the median arterial trunk is of no more than average proportions.

The artery of Adamkiewicz is at T.8 on the left side, but appears to be a relatively less important structure by virtue of the presence of many other collateral vessels.

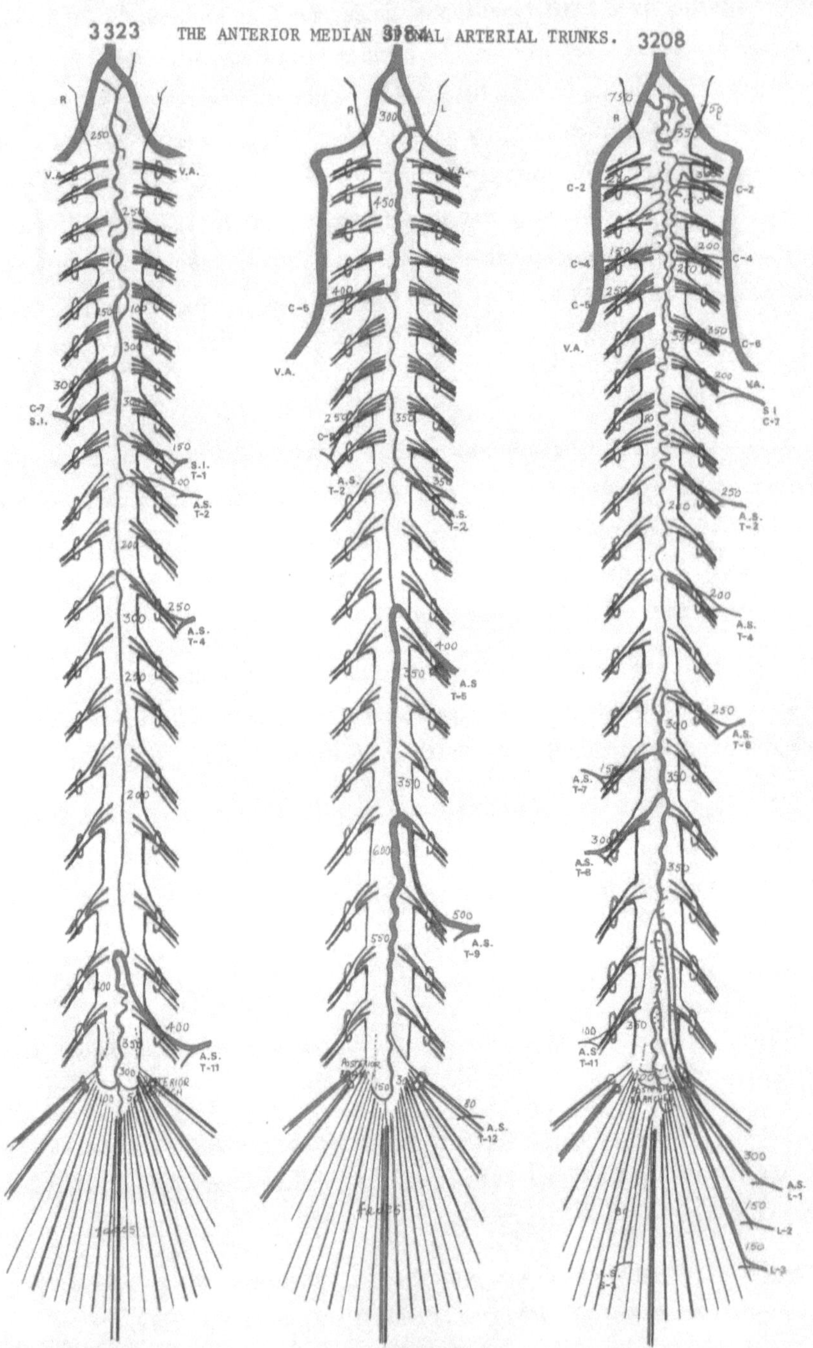

V.A. Vertebral Artery
A.C. Ascending Cervical Artery
D.C. Deep Cervical Artery
S.I. Superior Intercostal Artery
A.S. Aortic Segmental Artery (levels indicated)
I.L. ILIO–Lumbar Artery
L.S. Lateral Sacral Artery
The approximate size of the main arterial trunk and of each feeder vessel is indicated, in terms of micro–millimeters

PLATE 3

THE ANTERIOR MEDIAN ARTERIAL TRUNK OF THE SPINAL CORD (continued)

COMMENT ON PLATE IV

Cadaver 3247. In this specimen there are 2 arterial feeders only, the smallest number in the series. The well-spaced feeders at T.2 and T.8 levels, and their considerable sizes are sufficient to ensure the integrity of the anterior median arterial channel throughout its course in the thoracic region. In the event of injury to either of these feeders, the blood supply of the thoracic region could conceivably be compromised to the extent of leading to cord disturbance and partial or complete paraplegia.

At the distal extremity the well-developed posterior communicating vessels are displayed while in the filum terminale, the anterior median trunk diminishes in size and fades.

Cadaver 3212. This specimen would appear to enjoy a particularly robust blood supply, yet in the thoracic region the calibre of the anterior median trunk is of no more than average proportion.

Cadaver 3211. The most striking feature is the presence of a long, seemingly vulnerable section in the thoracic region. This is a common rather than an unusual finding, and once again stresses the fact that the vascularity of a part is in proportion to the normal needs, and not to abnormal demands such as may occur following injury or disease.

THE ANTERIOR MEDIAN SPINAL ARTERIAL TRUNKS.

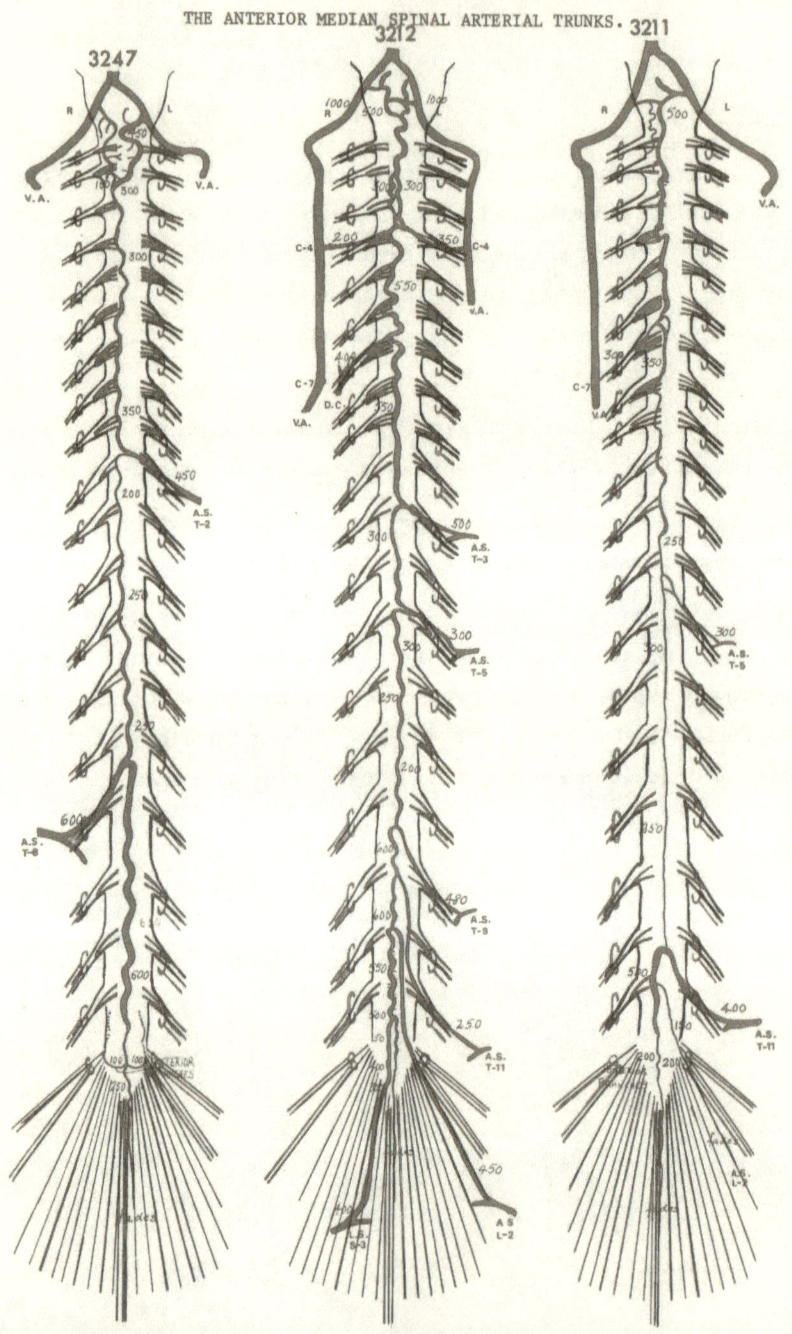

V.A. Vertebral Artery
A.C. Ascending Cervical Artery
D.C. Deep Cervical Artery
S.I. Superior Intercostal Artery
A.S. Aortic Segmental Artery (levels indicated)
I.L. ILIO-Lumbar Artery
L.S. Lateral Sacral Artery

The approximate size of the main arterial trunk and of each
feeder vessel is indicated, in terms of micro-millimeters

PLATE 4

THE ANTERIOR MEDIAN ARTERIAL TRUNK OF THE SPINAL CORD (continued)

COMMENT ON PLATE V

Cadaver 3296. The preponderance of arterial feeders from the vertebral artery is once again an obvious feature, and an unusually large number is present. (Refer also PLATE IX).

Over an extensive portion of the thoracic cord there is an absence of arterial feeders, and accordingly there is created a vulnerable zone which in the event of injury or disease could be associated with paraplegia. Surgical approaches to the vertebral bodies and to the anterior aspect of the cord must in all instances be governed in some measure by this factor, and when the spinal canal is at particular risk, there is a real indication for angiographic studies in advance of surgical procedures.

Cadaver 3303. There are arterial feeders at C.7 and T.1 levels on the left side, which are branches of the superior intercostal artery. In this series, the superor intercostal artery contributes only 5 out of a total of 62 arterial feeders to the cervical cord.

Cadaver 3328. At the distal extremity a number of very small arterial branches is present and supply the roots of the cauda equina. They arise from posterior communicating arteries. These small branches are a constant feature in well-injected, well-filled specimens.

The lateral sacral artery contributes substantial arterial feeders at S.2 level in cadavers 3296 and 3328.

THE ANTERIOR MEDIAN SPINAL ARTERIAL TRUNKS.

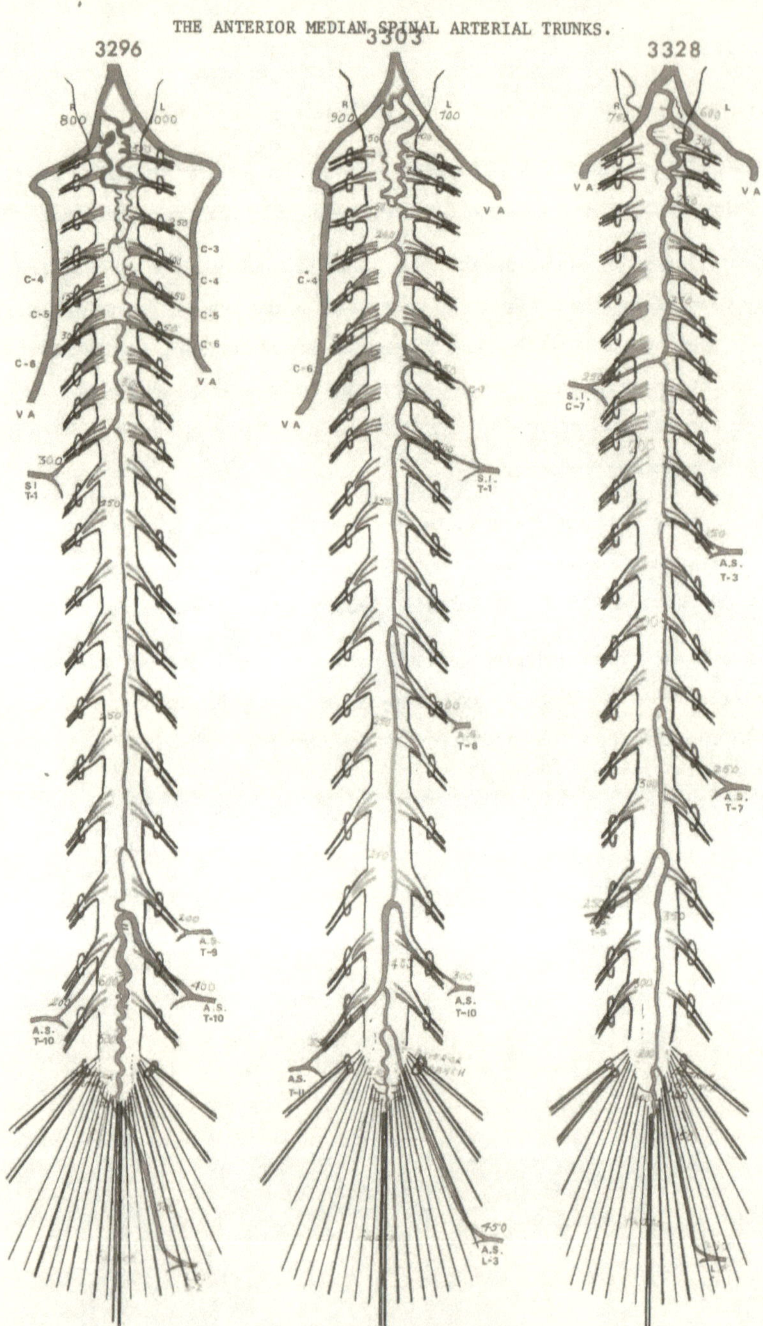

V.A.   Vertebral Artery
A.C.   Ascending Cervical Artery
D.C.   Deep Cervical Artery
S.I.   Superior Intercostal Artery
A.S.   Aortic Segmental Artery (levels indicated)
I.L.   ILIO—Lumbar Artery
L.S.   Lateral Sacral Artery

The approximate size of the main arterial trunk and of each
feeder vessel is indicated, in terms of micro—millimeters

PLATE   5

THE ANTERIOR MEDIAN ARTERIAL TRUNK OF THE SPINAL CORD (continued)

COMMENT ON PLATE VI

Duplication in whole or in part of the cervical anterior median arterial trunk is observed as a common feature.

In cadaver 3252, there are 3 cervical arterial feeders which arise from the deep cervical artery, an uncommon source in this series.

The variability of the individual patterns, and the consistency of the principle of a rich arterial system at cervical and lumbar enlargements, and a less rich system in the upper portion of the thoracic cord where the supply is in proportion to the demand, are factors which gain repeated emphasis.

The artery of Adamkiewicz is seen on the right side at T.10 level in specimen 3325.

In cadaver 3252, the lateral sacral artery contributes a reasonably substantial arterial feeder at L.5 level.

The spacing of the feeder vessels in the thoracic region, at the most advantageous positions for the supply of cord tissue at segmental levels remote from the points of entry of the feeders, and for the maintenance of the long arterial column is evident from even a super-ficial study of this set of diagrams.

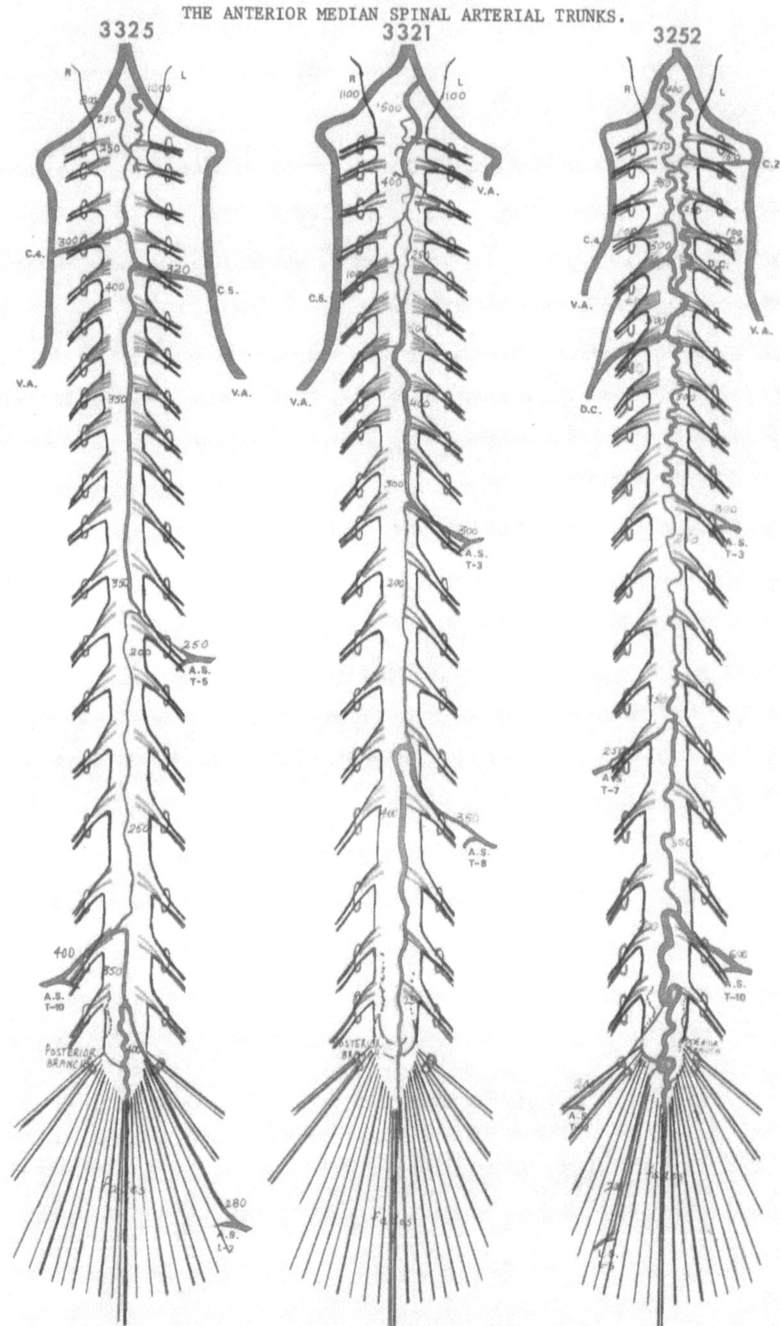

The approximate size of the main arterial trunk and of each
feeder vessel is indicated, in terms of micro—millimeters

THE ANTERIOR MEDIAN ARTERIAL TRUNK OF THE SPINAL CORD (continued

COMMENT ON PLATE VII

There is a striking demonstration of the principle that the blood supply is richest in the cervical and the lumbar regions where there are large ganglionic accumulations and where the metabolic demands are greatest. The constancy of size of the thoracic of the anterior median arterial trunk is also clearly demonstrated. It is adequate for the needs of the thoracic section of the cord where white rather than grey matter predominates. The flow of blood to the extended thoracic section is generally presumed to be from both a proximal and a distal direction.

Cadaver 3443 displays an unusual variation of the left vertebral artery which by-passes the transverse foramina of C.1 and C.2 vertebrae.

The posterior communicating arteries at the region of the conus, connecting the anterior median arterial trunk to the postero-lateral trunk on one side only in two of the three specimens, are indicated. The consistencies as well as the individual variations of pattern are evident.

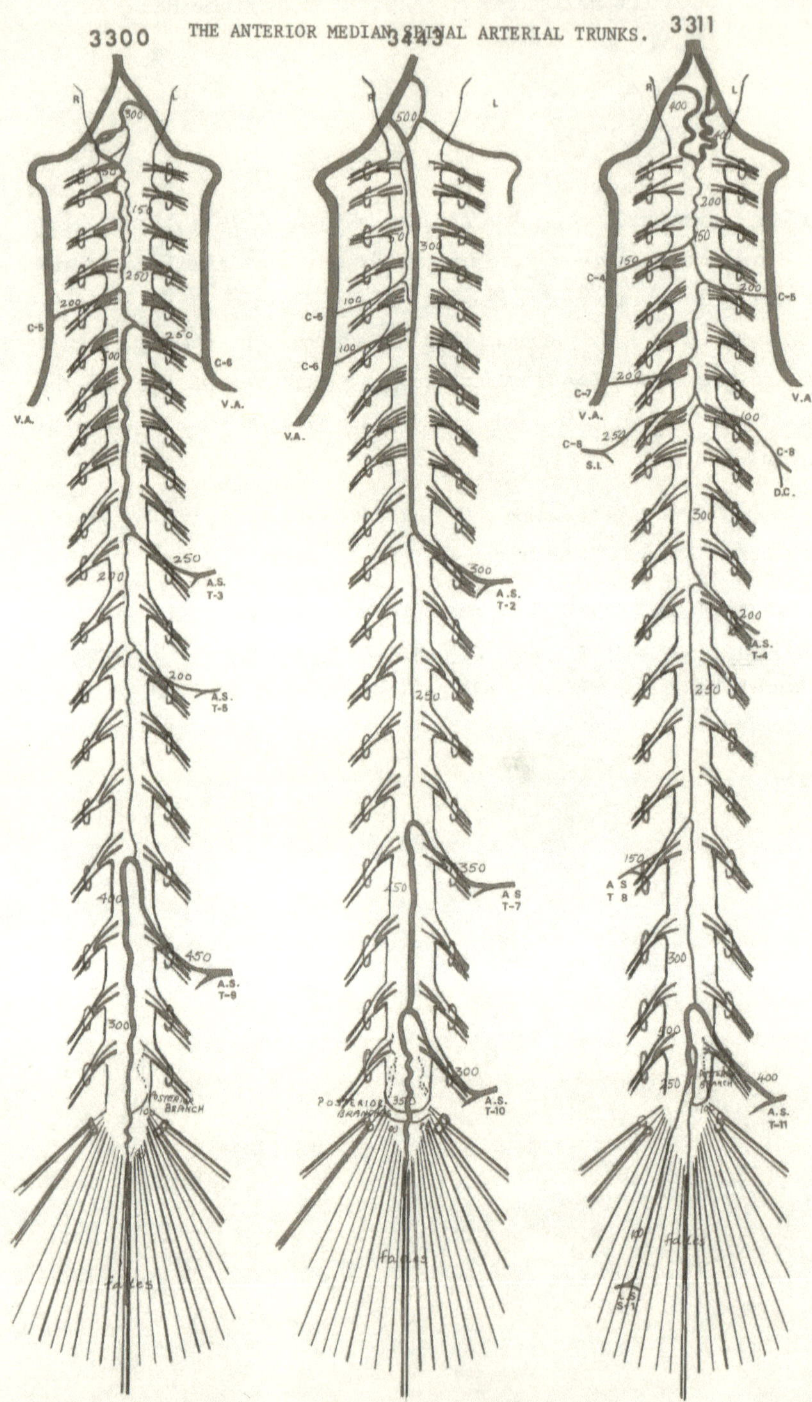

V.A. Vertebral Artery
A.C. Ascending Cervical Artery
D.C. Deep Cervical Artery
S.I. Superior Intercostal Artery

A.S. Aortic Segmental Artery (levels indicated)
I.L. ILIO—Lumbar Artery
L.S. Lateral Sacral Artery

The approximate size of the main arterial trunk and of each
feeder vessel is indicated, in terms of micro—millimeters

PLATE 7

THE ANTERIOR MEDIAN ARTERIAL TRUNK OF THE SPINAL CORD (continued)

The number of the arterial feeders, the location as to segmental level and to left/right sided incidence, and the approximate sizes are shown on PLATE VIII, overleaf. The artery of Adamkiewicz is indicated by the presence of a bar beneath the appropriate disc.

The total number of anterior arterial feeders (radicular arteries) in the series of 21 cadavers is 160, with an average of about 8 and with a variability of from 2-17. In 5 cases only, there are less than 3 and more than 10 arterial feeders. There is an over-all left-sided preponderance in the proportion of 3:2. There is a right-sided preponderance in the cervical region, of 3:2. In the cervical region, most feeders occur at C.4 - C.7 level. In the thoracic region, there are less than in the cervical and lumbar regions, but more than were expected from a perusal of the literature.

It is interesting to note that the heaviest thoracic incidence was at T.5 level, exactly halfway between the richly supplied cervical and lumbar regions, and at a point equidistant from the proximal and distal sources.

In the thoraco-lumbar region, from about T.8 to L.4 level, there is the heaviest concentration of large feeders, and in this area the artery of Adamkiewicz is encountered in the great majority of specimens. In this series, Adamkiewicz's artery occurred on the left side in 16 instances. In the sacral area there is only a light scatter of feeders, and in 7 specimens there is a feeder from the lateral sacral artery.

At the proximal extremity, communications between the median arterial trunk and the vertebral arteries occur in all instances, bilaterally in 16 cadavers and unilaterally in 5 cadavers. If the respective sizes of these channels is an indication of the direction of blood flow, then a variability of direction is detectable in the series (Refer Plate I, cadaver 3436 in which the median trunk is discontinuous. Refer Plate 2 Cadaver 3288, Plate 3 cadaver 3184, and Plate 6 cadaver 3252, in which the size of the median trunk diminishes as it proceeds in a cephalic direction. Refer Plate 2 cadaver 3292, in which an arterial circle appears to be present between the 2 vertebral arteries and a strong connecting vessel).

At the distal extremity, the anterior median arterial trunk communicates in the region of the conus medullaris with the postero-lateral arterial trunks by means of posterior communicating vessels which are present bilaterally in 13 instances and unilaterally in 6 instances. They were absent or unfilled and therefore not detectable in 2 instances.

The presence of small branches for the nourishment of the roots of the cauda equina was a constant feature when the vessels were well filled, and is indicated in Plate 5, cadavers 3296, 3303 and 3328. The anterior median arterial trunk as well as the 2 postero-lateral

THE FEEDER ARTERIES OF SUPPLY
of
The Anterior Median Arterial Trunk of the Spinal Cord

SEGM. LEVEL

R — CERVICAL — L

R — THORACIC — L

R — LUMBAR — L

R — SACRAL — L

Denotes vessel size 350 micro-millimeters or larger.

" " " 160 – 340 micro-millimeters.

" " " 20 – 150 " "

" Artery of Adamkiewicz.

trunks were studied in the same cadavers in 3 instances (Plate III cadaver 3208, Plate IV cadaver 3247 and Plate VI cadaver 3252).

It was not possible to establish a constant relationship between the two groups. In cadaver 3208, there were 17 anterior and 9 posterior arterial feeders, (radicular arteries), and the sum of the diameters of the set of anterior feeders amounted to 3830 micro-millimeters as compared with 1400 in the case of the posterior group.

In cadaver 3247 the relative numbers and total diameters were 2 anterior and 6 posterior vessels, and 1050 and 1000 micro-millimeters respectively.

In cadaver 3252 the relative numbers and total diameters were 10 anterior and 10 posterior vessels, and 2850 and 2050 micro-millimeters respectively. The numbers of anterior feeder vessels in each of the 21 cadavers in the series was as follows:

Number of anterior arterial feeders	Number of specimens in group	Specimen numbers
2	1	3247
3	2	3211. 3321
4	2	3301. 3323
5	3	3300. 3328. 3443
6	3	3184. 3325. 3444
7	Nil	
8	2	3303. 3436
9	2	3212. 3311
10	2	3288. 3252
12	1	3296
13	1	3447
14	1	3447
15	1	3292
17	1	3208
TOTAL	21	

Arterial feeders for the cervical cord arise predominantly from the vertebral artery. (Plate IX).

THE CERVICAL PORTION
of
The Anterior Median Arterial Trunk of the Spinal Cord

S p e c i m e n   N u m b e r — R

CERVICAL / THORACIC segmental levels. Feeder vessel codes: VA = vertebral artery, DC = deep costal, SI = superior intercostal, AC = ascending cervical, AS 2 = proximal aortic segmental artery.

SEGM. LEVEL	3443	3300	3311	3252	3321	3325	3328	3303	3296	3212	3211	3247	3208	3184	3323	3301	3292	3288	3447	3436	3444
CERVICAL																					
1																					
2													VA								
3																					
4			VA	VA		VA		VA	VA				VA					AC	VA		
5	VA	VA		VA	VA			VA	VA				VA	VA	VA	VA	VA	VA	VA		
6	VA							VA	VA	VA	VA							AC	VA	VA	
7			SI	DC			SI			DC					SI	VA	VA	VA	VA		VA
8			SI					SI						AS 2						SI	
THORACIC																					
1									SI												

S p e c i m e n   N u m b e r — L

SEGM. LEVEL	3444	3436	3447	3266	3292	3301	3323	3184	3208	3247	3211	3212	3296	3303	3328	3325	3321	3252	3311	3300	3443
CERVICAL																					
1																					
2								VA													
3		VA	VA																		
4					VA							VA	VA								
5			VA	VA	VA			VA			VA	VA	VA			VA	DC	VA			
6				VA	VA			VA					VA				VA	VA			
7							SI						SI								
8																		DC	DC		
THORACIC																					
1													SI								

The vertebral Artery provides 49 out of 62 feeder vessels in this series.
The Deep Costal and the Superior Intercostal Arteries each provide 5
feeder vessels, and the Ascending Cervical Artery provides 2 feeder vessels.
The proximal aortic segmental artery provides one vessel.
The Superior Intercostal Artery provides 3 feeder arteries at T.I segmental
level.

THE ANTERIOR MEDIAN ARTERIAL TRUNK OF THE SPINAL CORD (continued)
The photographic appearances of the length of the anterior aspect of the spinal cord and
anterior vessels are reproduced. (Refer also Plate III, Cadaver 3208).

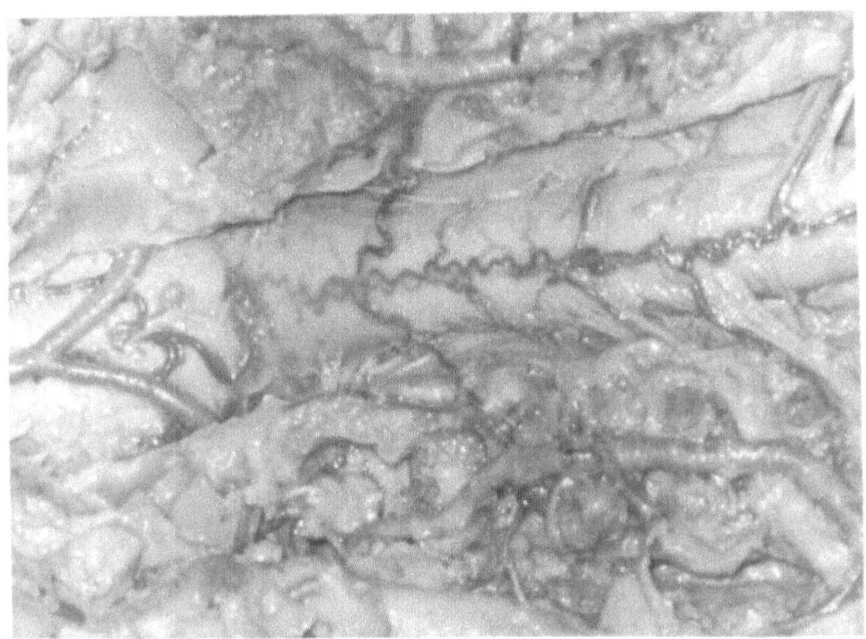

Fig. 5.   Cadaver 3208. The Anterior median arterial trunk from proximal extremity to
C.6 level. Feeder arteries at C.2 & C.6 on the left and at C.2, 4 & 5 levels on
the right side. A radicular vessel accompanies C.3 nerve root on the right side.
(x16)

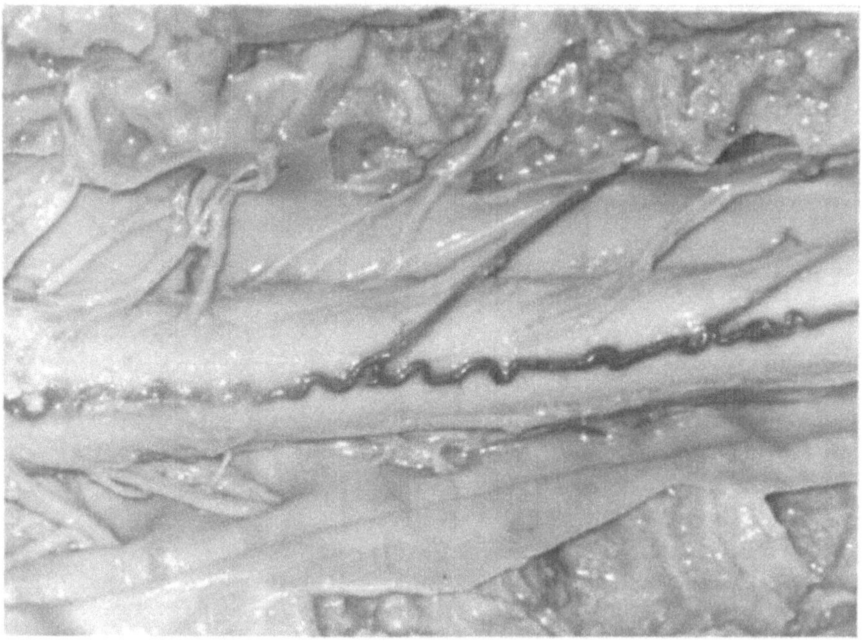

Fig. 6.   Cadaver 3208. The anterior median arterial trunk at C.7 – T.4, with feeders
at T.2 & 4 on the left side. (x16)

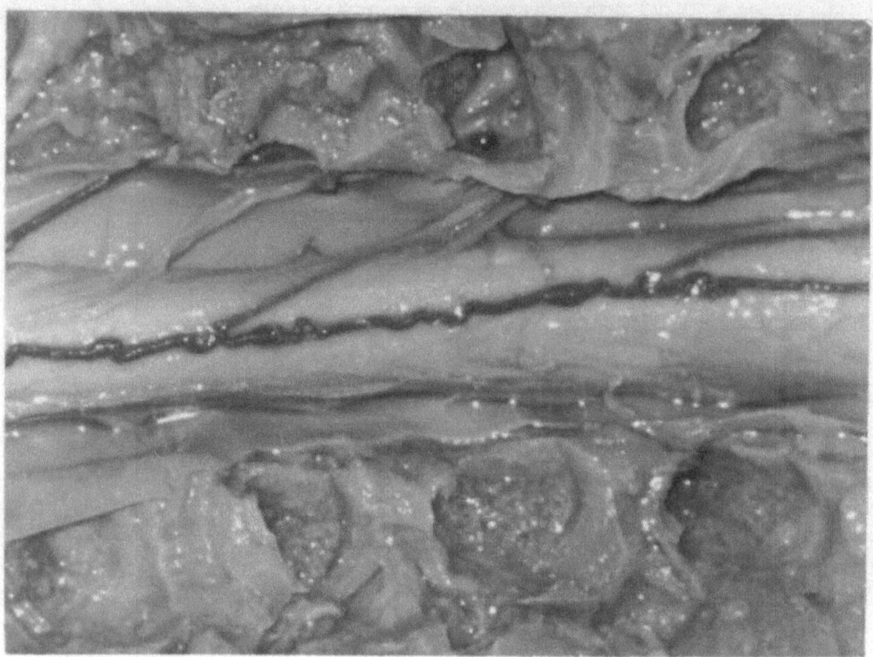

Fig. 7.   Cadaver 3208. The anterior median arterial trunk at T.2 – T.6 level with feeder vessels at T.2 & T.4 on the left side. (x16).

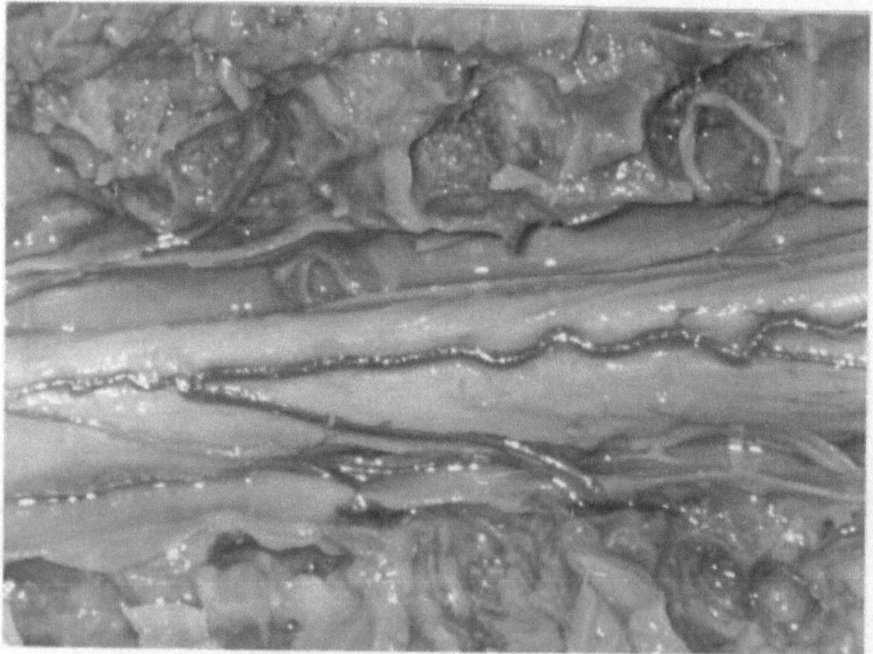

Fig. 8.   Cadaver 3208. The anterior median arterial trunk at T.6 – T.10, with feeder vessels at T.6 on the left and at T.7 & T.8 on the right side. The stumps of the vertebral pedicles are seen on the left side, at the top of the field. (x16).

THE ANTERIOR MEDIAN ARTERIAL TRUNK OF THE SPINAL CORD (continued)

INTERRUPTION OF THE ANTERIOR MEDIAN TRUNK was encountered in 2 specimens in the series (Fig. 10; also PLATE 1 cadaver 3436). In each instance, the termination of the arterial trunk took the form of a break-down into a number of smaller vessels which entered the median sulcus and became reduced in size to dimensions beyond the scope of this investigation. (Fig. 19, cadaver 3447).

THE ANTERIOR SPINAL ARTERY, which forms a communication at the proximal level of the anterior median trunk with the vertebral artery occurs unilaterally in 5 out of 21 specimens in the series. In no instance was total absence of this communicating vessel recorded. (Ref. Plate 1 and others).

DUPLICATION OF THE ANTERIOR MEDIAN TRUNK in the cervical region occurred in 13 cadavers (Fig. XI cadaver 3436). The duplication was confined to a short section in some cases and was more extensive in others. It is the result of failure of fusion, in whole or in part, of the paired embryonal anterior vessels, and is associated with no apparent advantage over the single vessel.

THE PERFORATING ARTERIES OF THE MEDIAN SULCUS displayed a pattern in close fulfulment of the principle of a rich blood supply where the demand is greatest, namely at the cervical and the lumbar enlargements of the cord, (Figs. 12, 13, 17 and 18), and a less rich supply in the upper segments of the thoracic cord in which there is no neural enlargement, (Figs. 14, 15 and 16). At the conus medullaris, (Fig. 9; Fig. 18), the perforating vessels are large and numerous. It is at this area also that the communicating vessels pass from the anterior to the postero-lateral arterial trunks. It may therefore be seen as a highly complex region in which the lumbar enlargement of the cord is found together with an arterial plexus and the roots of the cauda equina. It is placed at the junction of the immobile and the mobile parts of the vertebral column, an area prone to trauma. It is in this area that 'root escape', so named by Holdsworth and Hardy (1953), is seen in a substantial proportion of fractures and fracture-dislocations.

THE ARTERY OF ADAMKIEWICZ.

Adamkiewicz (1882) described the large feeder which occurs in the lower thoracic or in the lumbar area as the 'arteria radicalis anterior magna'. In this series, it occurs on the left side in 16 specimens, on the right side in 4 specimens, and is absent in one specimen. It was found in 15 instances at T.8 - T.11 level, and in 5 at L.2 - L.4 level. The most common single level at which it occurred was T.11, in 5 cases.

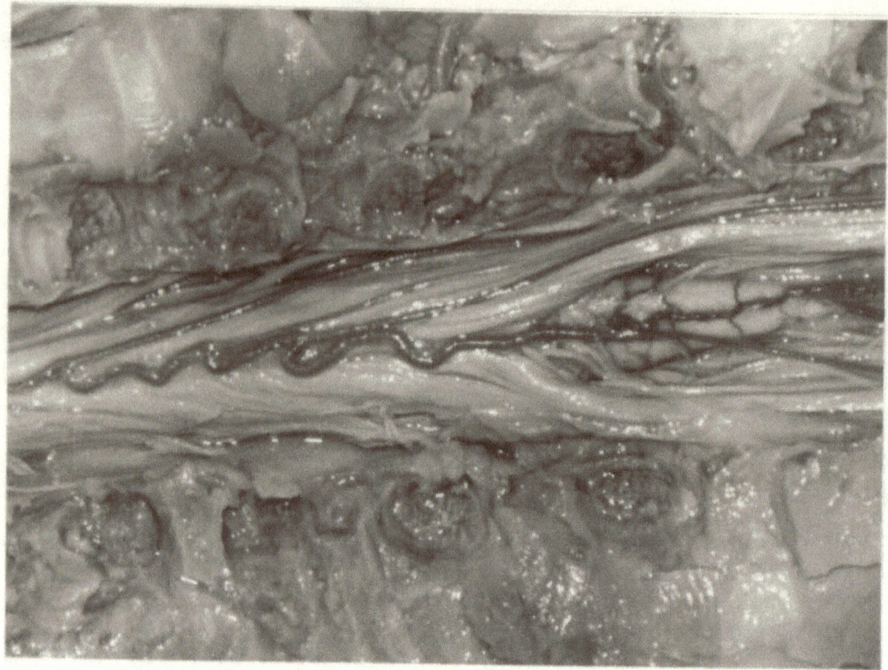

Fig. 9. Cadaver 3208. The anterior median trunk of the cord at T.10–conus medullaris level, with arterial feeder vessels at L.1,2 & L.3 on the left, and a small feeder at T.11 on the right side. (x16).

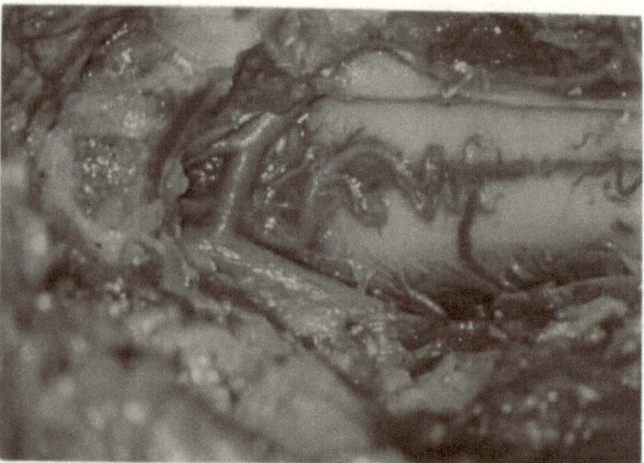

Fig. 10. Cadaver 3436. The anterior median arterial trunk at its proximal extremity, with communications extending to the vertebral artery on the left side only, and with a discontinuous median trunk at the level of C.2 roots. (x16).

THE ANTERIOR MEDIAN ARTERIAL TRUNK OF THE SPINAL CORD

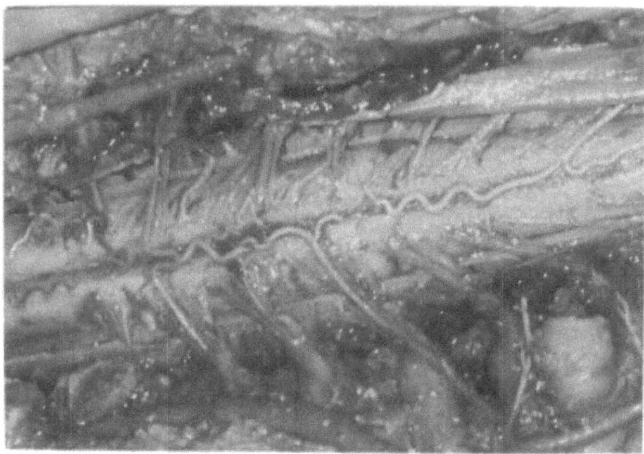

Fig. 11   Cadaver 3436. The spinal cord 'in situ' at C.3-T.1 level, with feeder arteries arising from the vertebral arteries which are displayed on both sides. (x10).

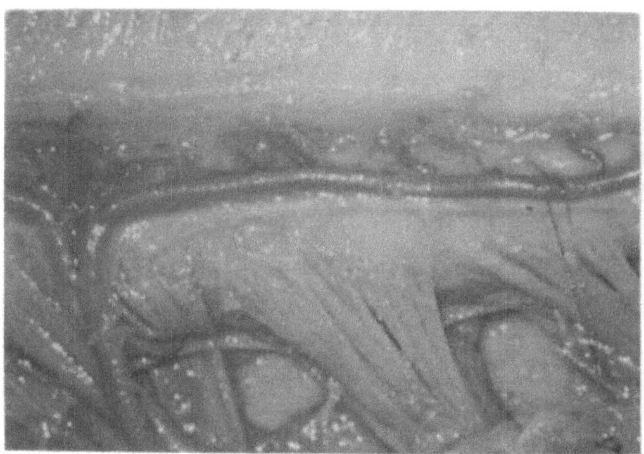

Fig. 12.   Cadaver 3447. The anterior median sulcus of the cord at C.7-T.1 level, with multiple central perforating arteries entering at the sulcus for the supply of the cord. (x25).

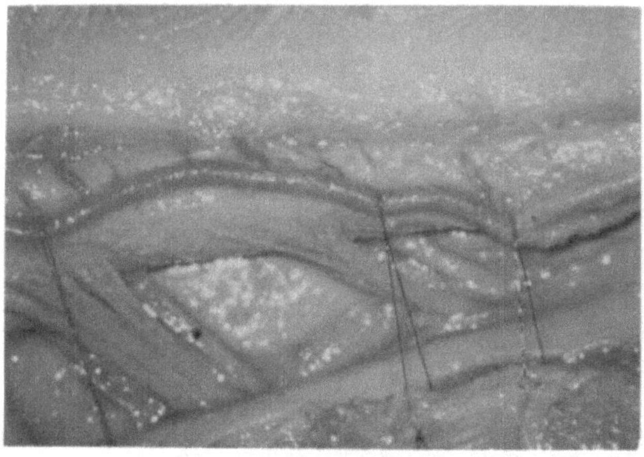

Fig. 13.   Cadaver 3447. The perforating arteries of the anterior median sulcus of the cord are numerous at T.1 level, and are diminishing in number and size at T.2. (x25).

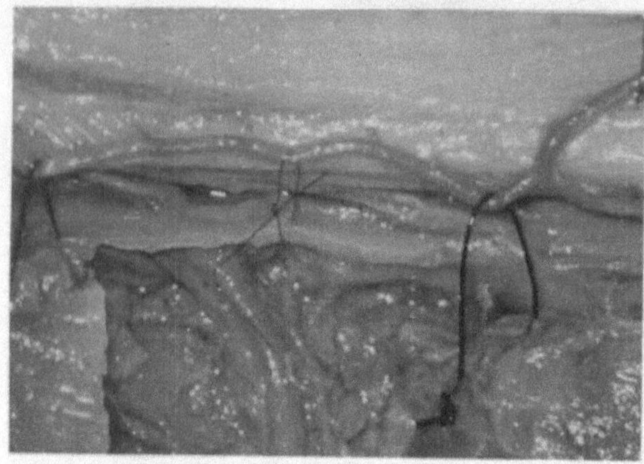

Fig. 14.   Cadaver 3447. The anterior median arterial trunk is retracted to display the perforating sulcal arteries at T.5 level, where they are found at about 1 cm. intervals
and where filling is poor on account of their small size. (x25)

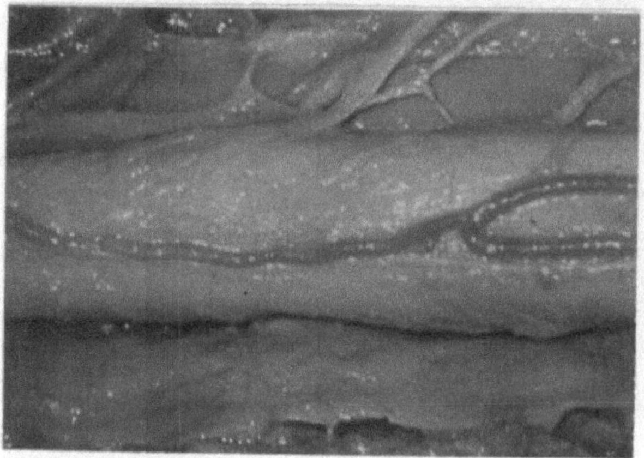

Fig. 15.   Cadaver 3447. The anterior median arterial trunk at T.6–T.7, showing the absence
of sulcal vessels of sufficient calibre to be filled by the technique employed. (Less
than 20 micro-millimeters).

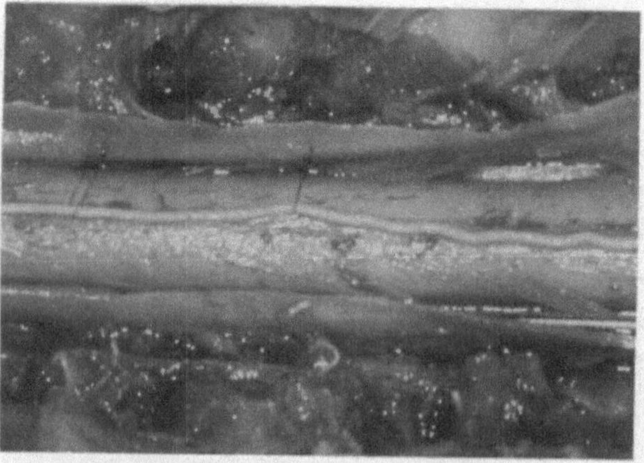

Fig. 16.   Cadaver 3436. The anterior median arterial trunk at T.8–T.10 level, where the
perforating sulcal arteries are too small to be demonstrated. (x16).

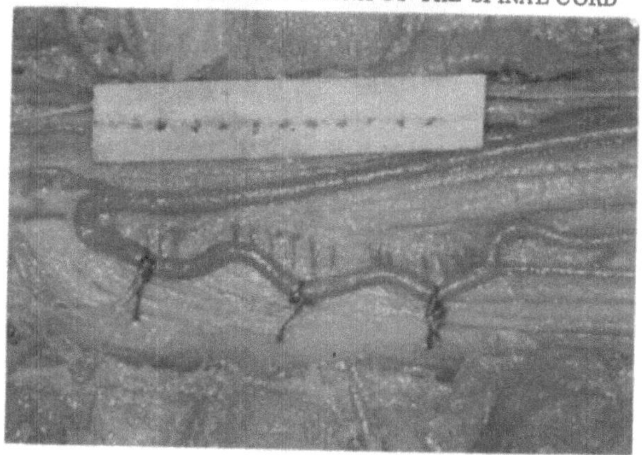

Fig. 17.   Cadaver 3447. The anterior median sulcus at T.12–L.1 level, with multiple perforating sulcal arteries. There are approximately 15 within the space of 1 cm. (x25).

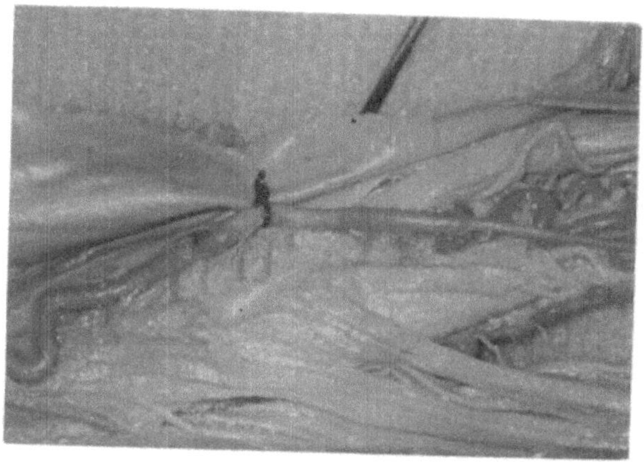

Fig. 18.   Cadaver 3252. The distal extremity of the anterior median arterial trunk, with multiple perforating sulcal arteries in the region of the conus. (x25).

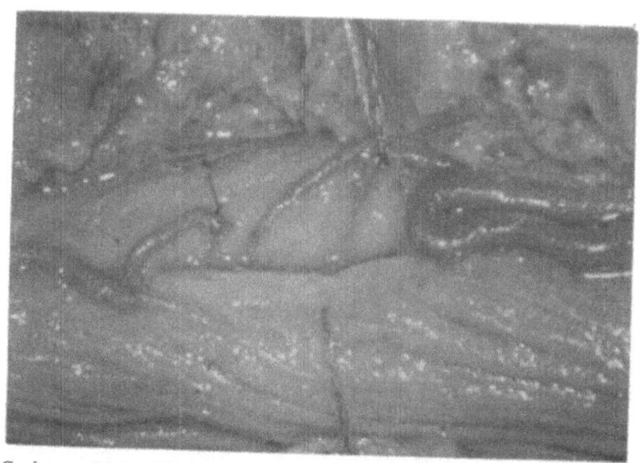

Fig. 19.   Cadaver 3447. The anterior arterial trunk in this specimen is interrupted at T.12–L.1 level, where it terminates in the median sulcus. The green thread is approximately 200 microns. (x25).

THE ANTERIOR MEDIAN ARTERIAL TRUNK OF THE SPINAL CORD (continued)

ARTERIO-ARTERIAL ANASTOMOSES

The presence of arterial anastomoses, also referred to elsewhere as "arterial by-passes", and "substitution pathways", and "loops", and "circles", are common at all levels of the verte- bral column, from the occipito-cervical junction to the sacrum. They occur also in struc- tures unrelated to the vertebrae, eg. in the muscle of the tongue between the lingual and the superior thyroid arteries, and in the thyroid gland parenchyma.

Proximo-distally, a number of anastomoses are illustrated (figs. 3, 20, 22, 23, 24, 25, 26).

In the cervical region, there are numerous anastomoses between descending branches of the ascending pharyngeal artery, and branches from the vertebral and ascending cervical arteries.

The deep cervical artery undoubtedly makes similar contributions but they have not been specifically sought. The superior intercostal artery and the most proximal of the aortic segmental arteries in the thoracic region communicate by arterial loops, and at various levels in various cadavers, anastomoses are found between segmental arteries and their ad- jacent companions.

In the lumbar and sacral regions, there are numerous anastomoses involving the lumbar seg- mental arteries, the ilio-lumbar, lateral sacral and the median sacral arteries. In addition, there is at every segmental level a transverse arterial arch of communication between the left and right segmental arteries, passing across the anterior aspect of the dural sac within the extra-dural space and supplying nutrient vessels to the vertebral bodies by means of a number of branches which perforate the posterior longitudinal ligament. In addition, they supply numerous small vessels to the dura which in the human infant is a richly vascularised structure.

THE ANTERIOR MEDIAN ARTERIAL TRUNK OF THE SPINAL CORD.

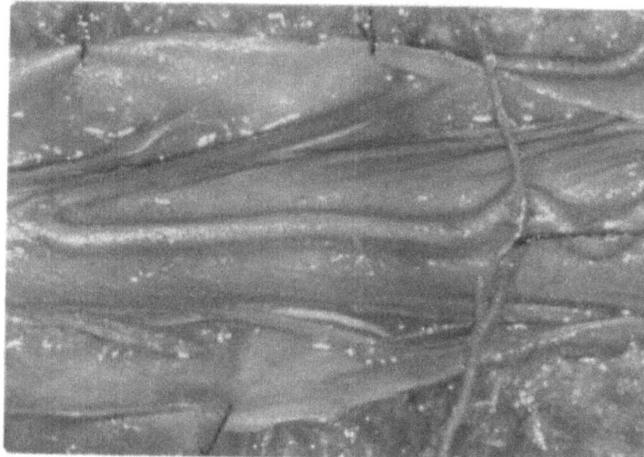

Fig. 20. Cadaver 3185. The artery of Adamkiewicz on the left side at T.11. It enters the sub-dural space by penetrating the dural membrane, where it could suffer constriction. (x25).

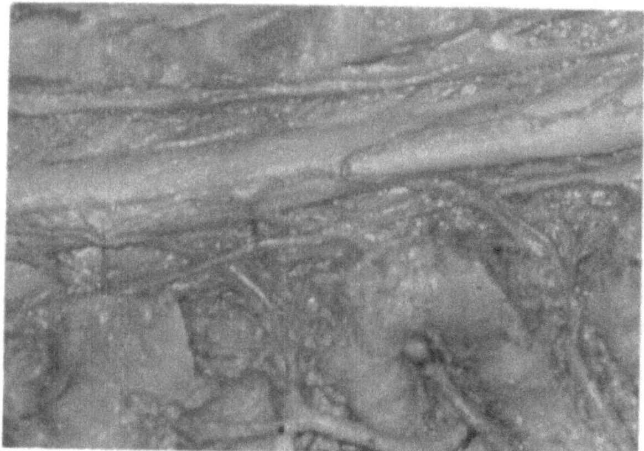

Fig. 21. Cadaver 3447. The anterior median artery at T.1-T.7. Arterial feeders arise from the segmental aortic thoracic arteries. The narrow zone of the spinal canal which normally covers 4-5 segments is apparent. (x16).

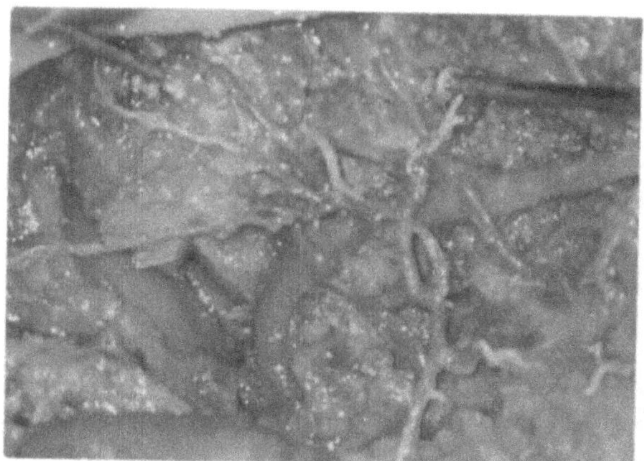

Fig. 22. Cadaver 3326. The vertebral artery turns to enter the foramen of C.1 transverse process. Arterio-arterial anastomoses occur between branches of the vertebral, the ascending cervical and the ascending pharyngeal arteries. (x25).

THE ANTERIOR MEDIAN ARTERIAL TRUNK OF THE SPINAL CORD.

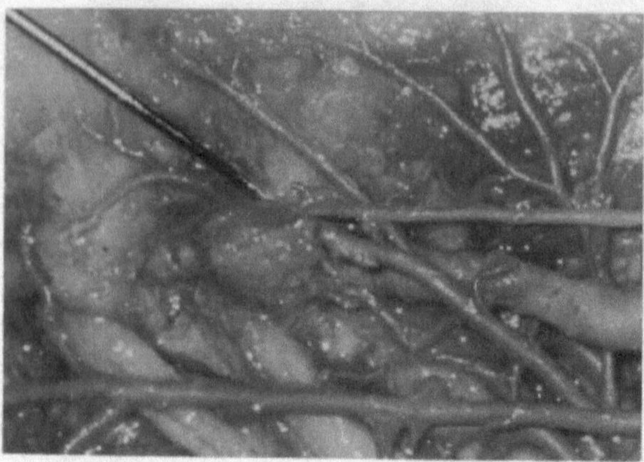

Fig. 23. Cadaver 3212. Arterio-arterial anastomoses, between an unnamed branch of the subclavian artery and the vertebral artery at C.5-C.6, within the transverse foramen. (x16).

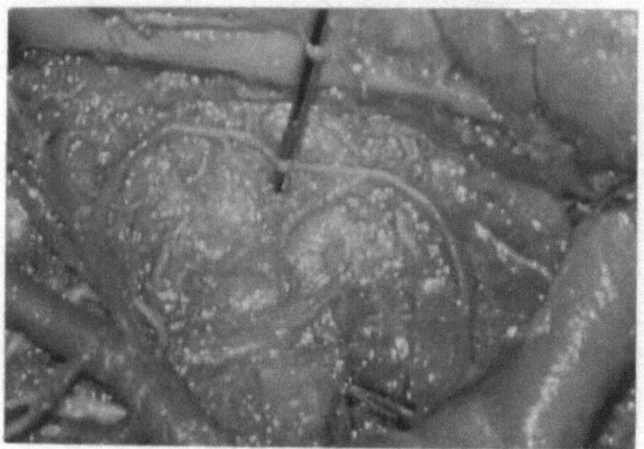

Fig. 24. Cadaver 3326. An arterio-arterial anastomoses between a branch of the superior intercostal artery and one from the most proximal segmental branch of the thoracic aorta. (x25).

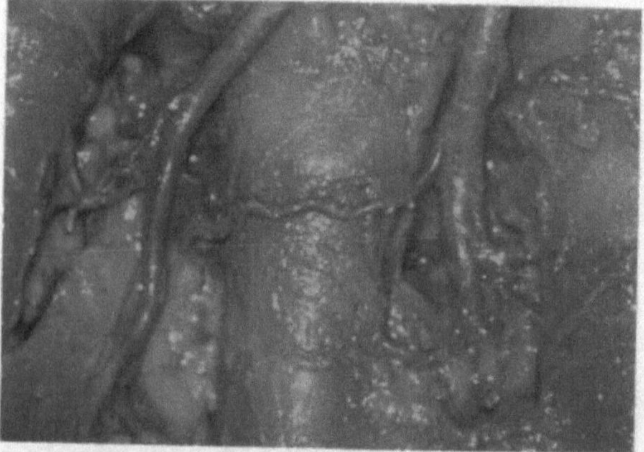

Fig. 25. Cadaver 3212. An arterio-arterial anastomoses between two adjacent aortic segmental arteries in the thorax. (x25).

THE ANTERIOR MEDIAN ARTERIAL TRUNK OF THE SPINAL CORD

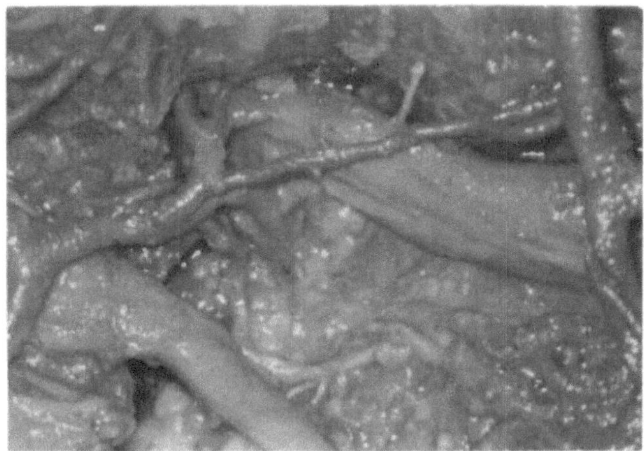

Fig. 26. Cadaver 3212. An arterio-arterial anastomoses is present, between the 12th
thoracic and the 1st lumbar aortic segmental arteries. The nerve roots of T.12
and L.1 emerge from the inter-vertebral foramina. (x25).

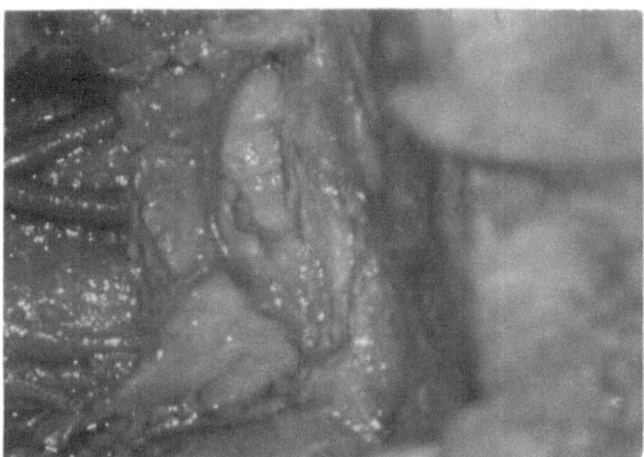

Fig. 27. Cadaver 3447. An arterial anastomoses or 'arcade' which crosses from side to
side across the anterior aspect of the dural sac at the lower thoracic level.
From this arcade, there arise nutrient arteries for the vertebral body, which
penetrate the posterior longitudinal ligament. Branches are given off for the
dural sac also. At the left of the field the dura has been divided and partially
removed to expose the cord with the anterior median arterial trunk and a large
arterial feeder. (x25).

THE POSTERO-LATERAL ARTERIAL TRUNKS OF THE SPINAL CORD

Two arterial trunks extend from the cephalic end of the cord where they communicate with the posterior inferior cerebellar or the vertebral arteries, to the distal end where they communicate with the anterior trunk by means of short posterior communicating vessels in the region of the conus medullaris. The number, location and relative sizes of the posterior arterial feeders of 9 cadavers are indicated in Plate XI.

The posterior trunks and collaterals are smaller and more numerous than the anterior and are adequately filled by the injection medium in a relatively small number of cases. For this reason, and because they take the form of more tortuous channels with numerous branches and tributaries which diverge and converge, and which weave a course between the posterior rootlets of the spinal nerves, they are displayed in their entirety only with difficulty.

PLATE X. When the posterior nerve rootlets are divided at source and retracted laterally, then the longitudinal trunks and the short transverse communicating channels, (Fig. 35) are clearly demonstrated.

There are 120 posterior arterial feeders (radicular arteries) in the 9 cadavers of this series, the average number per cadaver being 13.3 as compared with 7, 6 in the anterior study - almost twice as many. The calibre of the posterior vessels is however considerably smaller and individual variations are from 6, (Cadaver 3247), to 22, (cadaver 3492).

The numerical incidence is as follows:

Number of Posterior Arterial feeders	Number of specimens in group	Specimen Numbers
6	1	3247
9	2	3208. 3326
10	1	3252
12	2	3457. 3446
16	1	3210
17	1	3254
22	1	3492

The source of origin of all posterior arterial feeders has been traced in specimen 3492, and has been found to resemble closely the source of the anterior feeders, namely, a predominance of vertebral artery branches in the cervical area, and of the segmental arteries at other levels which coincide with the levels of the feeders.

The junction between feeder vessels and longitudinal channels is Y-shaped in the cervical and thoracic regions, and "pulled up inverted U-shaped" in the thoraco-lumbar and lumbar regions, as in the case of the anterior feeders. The growth theory in regard to the junctions is supported by the similarity of configuration of the two groups of vessels.

THE POSTERO-LATERAL ARTERIAL TRUNKS OF THE SPINAL CORD (continued)

Posterior communicating arteries from the postero-lateral to the anterior median trunks were present in 7 of the series, and could not be detected in 2 cadavers. In 2 cadavers, there was a right-sided preponderance. In 4 cadavers, the left and right-sided communicating arteries were of equal proportions.

By contrast with the anterior arterial feeders there was a right-sided preponderance of the posterior vessels in the proportion of 5:4. The slight superiority in numbers on the right side persisted throughout the cervical, thoracic, lumbar and sacral regions.

In 3 instances, dissections were pursued of both the anterior and the posterior groups of feeders, and there was no evidence of a co-ordinated plan or formula which related the pattern of one group to the other.

COMMENT ON PLATE X

The dissections of the postero-lateral arterial trunks and their feeders are presented in diagrammatic form. In each case, there is a double trunk which is continuous on both sides.

The postero-lateral trunks and their feeders are of smaller calibre than their anterior counterparts, but more numerous.

As in the case of the anterior system of vessels, there is a more profuse arterial supply in the region of the cervical and lumbar enlargements, and a less rich supply to the thoracic cord. Numerous transverse communicating channels connect the two trunks in the cervical and the lumbar regions. Proximally there is a well-defined communication with the inferior cerebellar artery or with the vertebral artery. Distally, there are communications on one or both sides with the anterior median trunk in the region of the conus. The Y-shaped junctions between feeders and longitudinal trunks in the cervical and thoracic regions are seen posteriorly as well as anteriorly. At the lumbar region, the inverted-U shape of the arterial junctions is the same as in the anterior system.

The distribution of the posterior feeder vessels is indicated in a 'scatter-gram', Plate XI.

THE POSTERO-LATERAL SPINAL ARTERIAL TRUNKS.

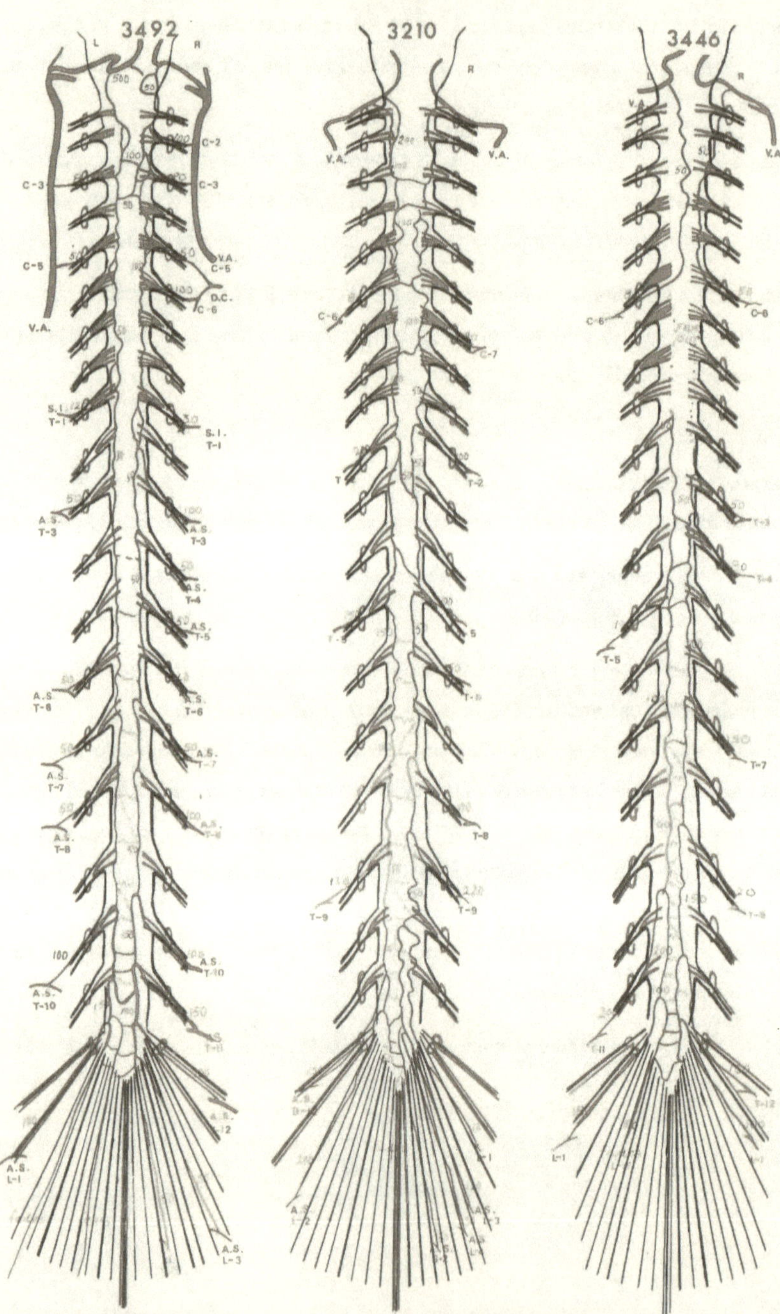

V.A. Vertebral Artery
A.C. Ascending Cervical Artery
D.C. Deep Cervical Artery
S.I. Superior Intercostal Artery

A.S. Aortic Segmental Artery (levels indicated)
I.L. ILIO-Lumbar Artery
L.S. Lateral Sacral Artery

The approximate size of the main arterial trunk and of each
feeder vessel is indicated, in terms of micro-millimeters

PLATE 10

THE FEEDER ARTERIES OF SUPPLY
of
The Postero-Lateral Arterial Trunks of the Spinal Cord.

Dot sizes follow the legend below: `●` = 200 µmm or larger; `●●` = 101–200 µmm; `•` = 51–100 µmm; `·` = 0–50 µmm.

3247	3208	3252	3254	3457	3326	3492	3446	3210	SEGMENTAL LEVEL	3210	3446	3492	3326	3457	3254	3252	3208	3247
			L						CERVICAL				R					
									1									
									2			•						
		●●				•			3			•						
					●●				4					●●				
		●				•			5				•	•		●		
	●●	●				•	•		6		•	•	●●	●				
					●●				7	●●					●			
									8								●●	
			L						THORACIC				R					
	•		●			●●			1			•			●			
●									2	•								
						·			3		•		●●			●		
·		●							4		•	•	●●					
				•	●●	•	●●		5	•		•		•			•	
									6			•				●		·
		●●	●						7						●			
					●●	·			8			•	●●	●●			●●	
	●●			●					9	●	●●							
						•			10					●●	●●	●		
				●●	●●		●●		11				●●				●●	
	●●		●			●●			12		●●	•					●●	
			L						LUMBAR				R					
			•			•	●●		1	●●	•			●●				●●
●						●●			2					•	●			●●
									3	●●			•					
									4	•			•					
		•	●	•		•			5					•	•			
			L						SACRAL				R					
					•				1					•	●			
									2	•								
			•						3				•					
									4									
		●							5									

●	Denotes vessel size 200 micro-millimeters or larger.
●●	" " " 101 - 200 micro-millimeters
•	" " " 51 - 100 "
·	" " " 0 - 50 " "

THE POSTERO-LATERAL ARTERIAL TRUNKS OF THE SPINAL CORD

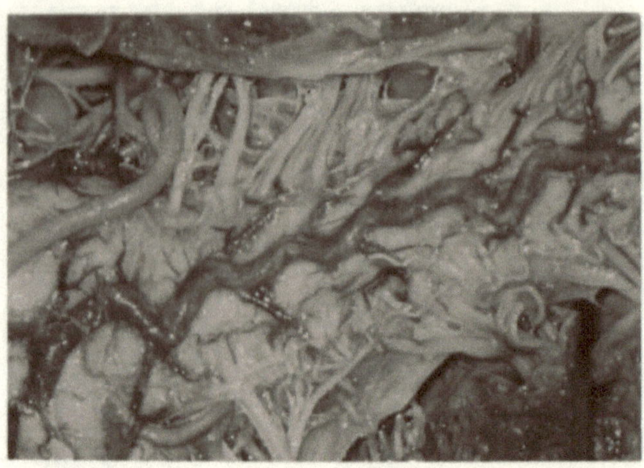

Fig. 28. Cadaver 3254. The postero-lateral arterial trunks of the spinal cord at C.1-C.4 level. The right posterior inferior cerebellar artery, (a large pink vessel at top left), communicates with the longitudinal trunk which is partly obscured by the posterior nerve rootlets. The left postero-lateral trunk is larger than the right. The large brown vessel which crosses the field from left to right is the longitudinal venous trunk which extends from the cranial cavity to the sacral region. It receives numerous tributaries 'en route'. (x16)

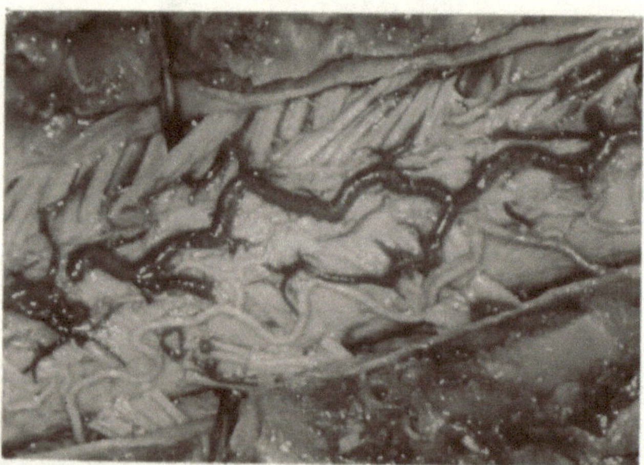

Fig. 29. Cadaver 3254. The posterior arterial trunks at C.6-T.1 level. The brown venous channel is filled with blood. The posterior nerve rootlets have been removed on the left side to expose the arterial trunk, which is obscured on the right side. (x16).

THE POSTERO-LATERAL ARTERIAL TRUNKS OF THE SPINAL CORD

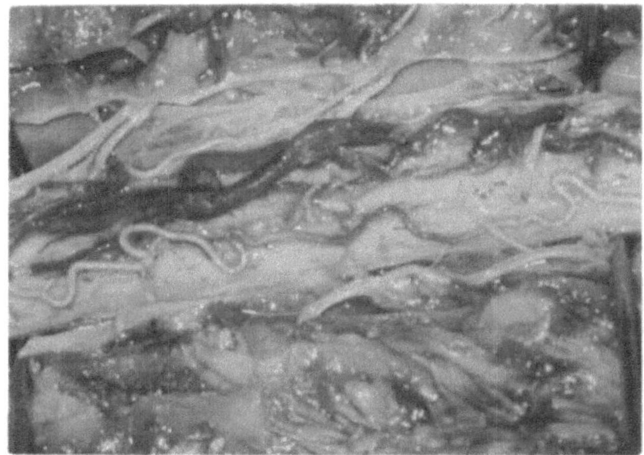

Fig. 30.   Cadaver 3254. The posterior arterial trunks at T.2-T.4 level. The median
venous channel pursues a wavy course. The arterial trunk on the left side
communicates with the opposite trunk via a number of small transverse
channels. (x16).

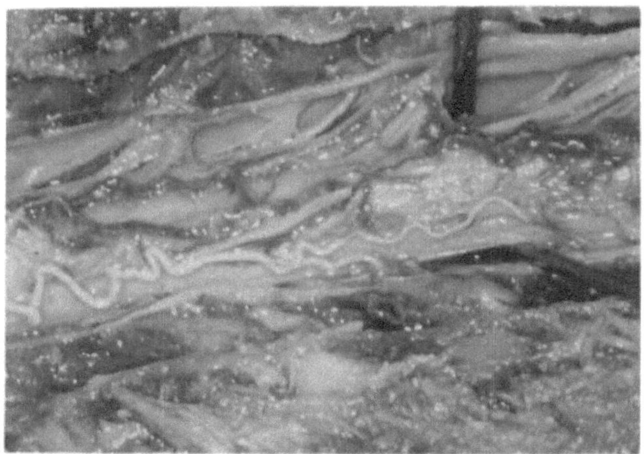

Fig. 31.   Cadaver 3254. The posterior arterial trunks at T.5-T.7 level. There are
feeder arteries at T.6 level on left and right sides. There is no break in
the continuity of the postero-lateral arterial channels. (x16).

THE POSTERO-LATERIAL ARTERIAL TRUNKS OF THE SPINAL CORD

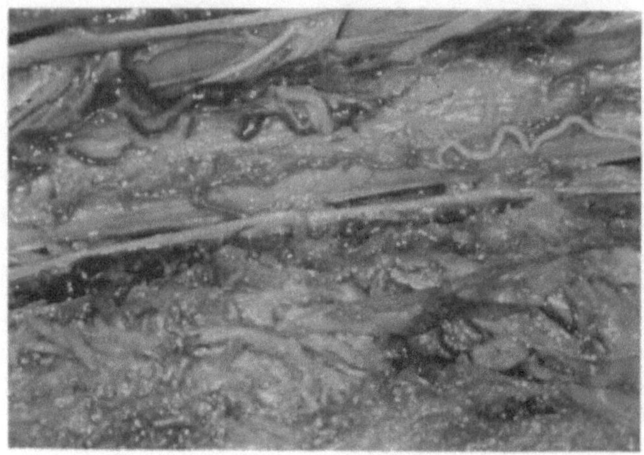

Fig. 32.   Cadaver 3254. The posterior arterial trunks at T.8 - T.10 level. Arterial filling is poor. A feeder vessel is present at T.9 level on the right side. (x16)

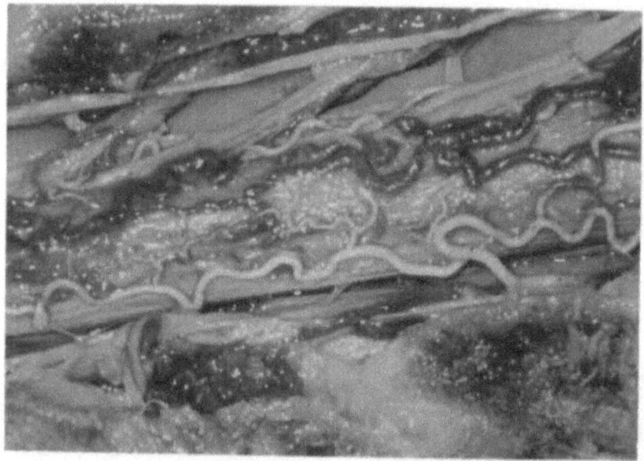

Fig. 33.   Cadaver 3254. As above, the posterior arterial trunks at T.11 - L.1 level. The nerve rootlets have been removed on the left side to display the continuity of the arterial trunk and the presence of transverse communicating vessels which connect the two trunks. The thickness of the dural membrane in the newborn is demonstrated, and the escaping nerve root is observed. (x16).

THE POSTERO–LATERAL ARTERIAL TRUNKS OF THE SPINAL CORD

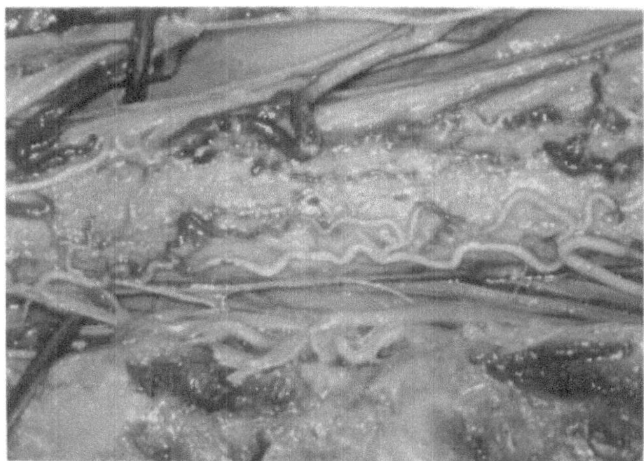

Fig. 34.   Cadaver 3254. The posterior arterial trunks are seen at thoraco–lumbar level.
There are large venous channels. There are numbers of transverse communicating channels between the two longitudinal trunks (x16).

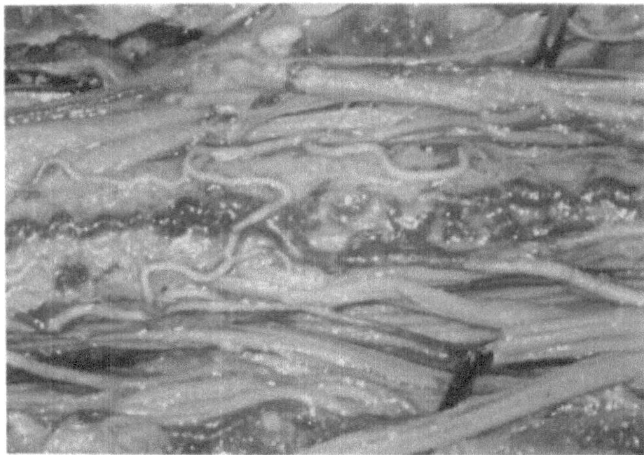

Fig. 35.   Cadaver 3254. The posterior channels at the distal end of the cord. The posterior nerve rootlets have been divided to expose the arterial trunks and communications. The metal 'retractors' have a diameter of 500 micro–millimeters.
The arteries are coloured pink and the veins which are filled with blood are
brown. (x16).

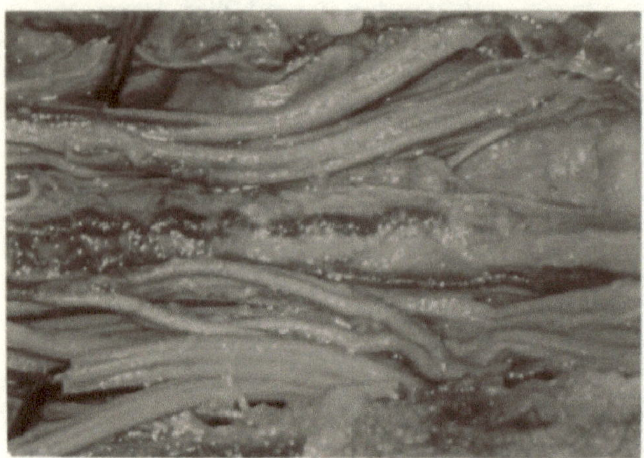

Fig. 36.   Cadaver 3254. The postero-lateral spinal arteries at the conus medullaris, with
the filum terminale. Feeder arteries accompany the nerve roots at L.2 and S.1
on the right side, and at S.5 level on the left side. (x16)

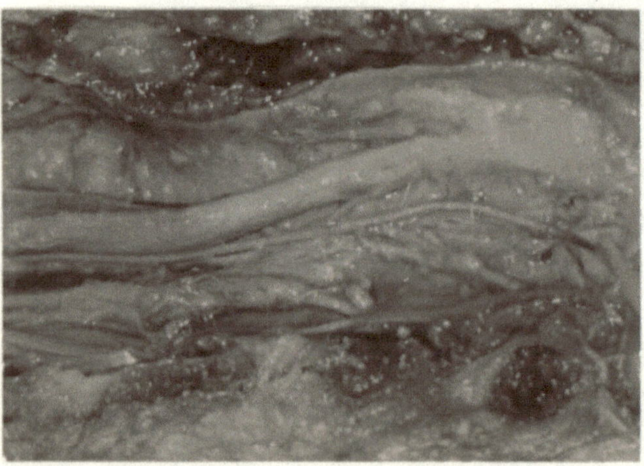

Fig. 37.   Cadaver 3254. The distal roots of the cauda equina are seen, and the spinal canal
at its distal extremity. An arterial feeder enters the canal at S.5 foramen on the
left side. (x16).

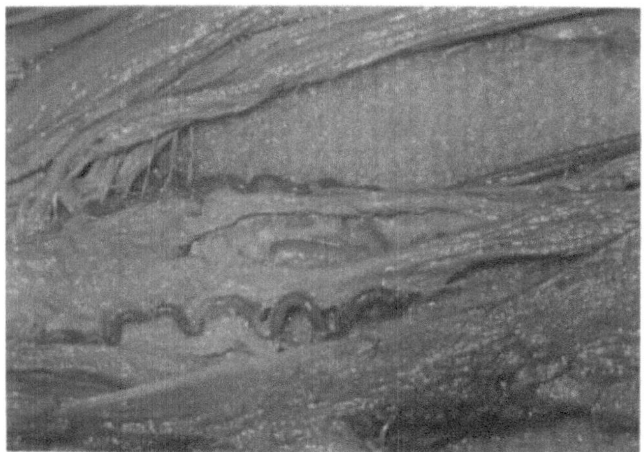

Fig. 38.   Cadaver 3252. The postero-lateral trunks are seen at the level of the conus medullaris, and a number of very small arteries for the supply of the roots of the cauda equina are nicely demonstrated. (x25).

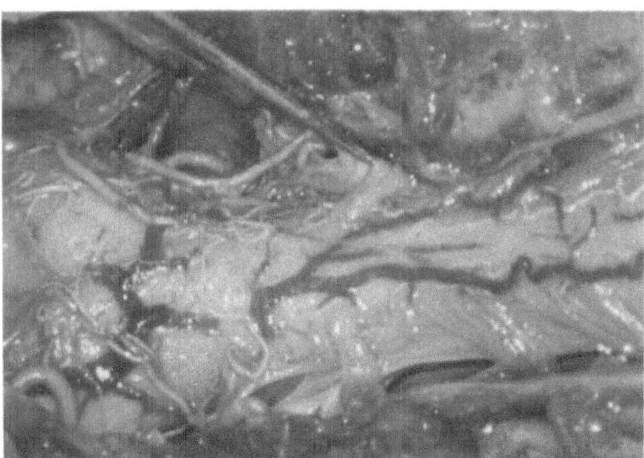

Fig. 39.   Cadaver 3492. The postero-lateral arterial trunks of the spinal cord at C.1–C.4 level. The medulla oblongata is at the left of the field where the posterior inferior cerebellar and the postero-lateral arterial trunks communicate via 'posterior spinal arteries'. The large brown venous channel which crosses the field is filled with blood. (x16).

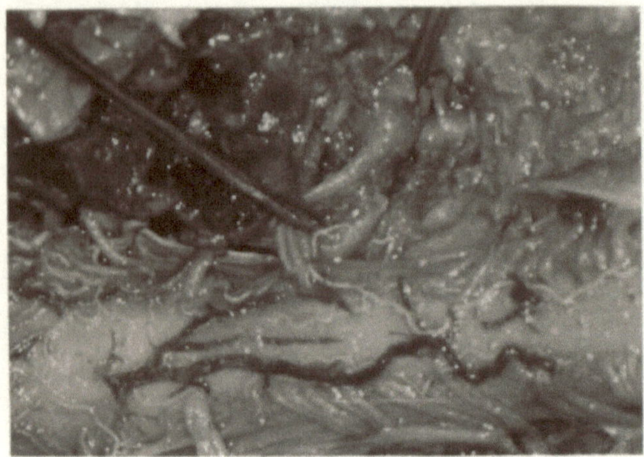

Fig. 40.   Cadaver 3492. The postero-lateral trunks at the proximal level of the cord, where a feeder vessel which accompanies the 2nd cervical nerve root on the right side, is shown arising from the vertebral artery within the transverse foramen. (x16).

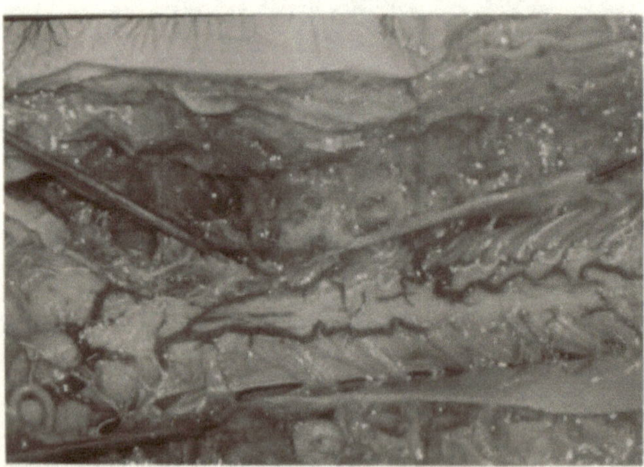

Fig. 41.   Cadaver 3492. The postero-lateral arterial trunks are partly obscured by the nerve rootlets on the left and right sides. The medulla oblongata is seen at left and the C.8 roots are seen on the right of the field. Observe the thick edges of the cut dural membrane. (x10).

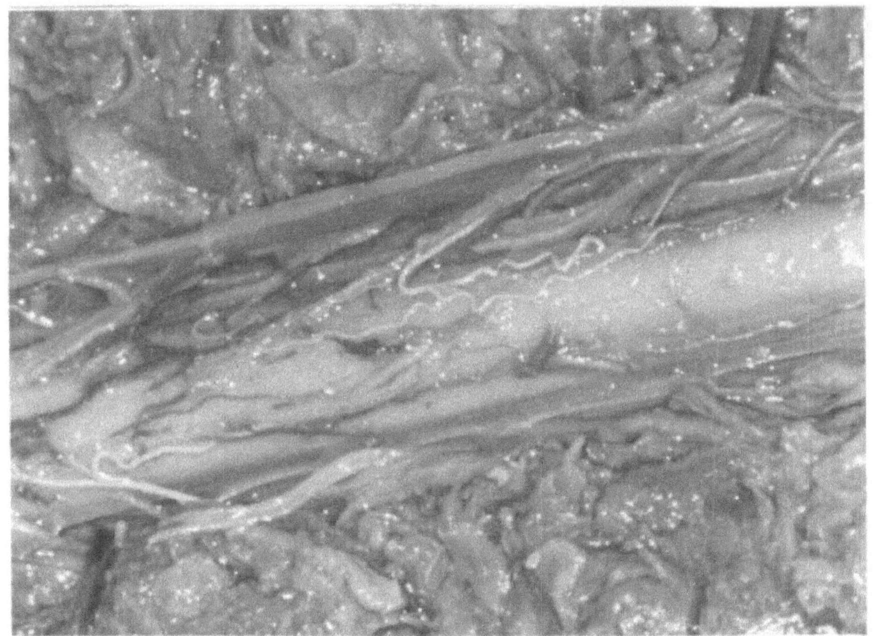

Fig. 42.   Cadaver 3492. The posterior arterial trunks at T.1–T.5 level. Feeder arteries
            are observed at T.1 on the right and at T.3, 4 and 5 levels on the left side. The
            thick cut edge of the dural membrane, and the almost transparent pial membrane
            with the dentate ligaments are clearly displayed. (x16)

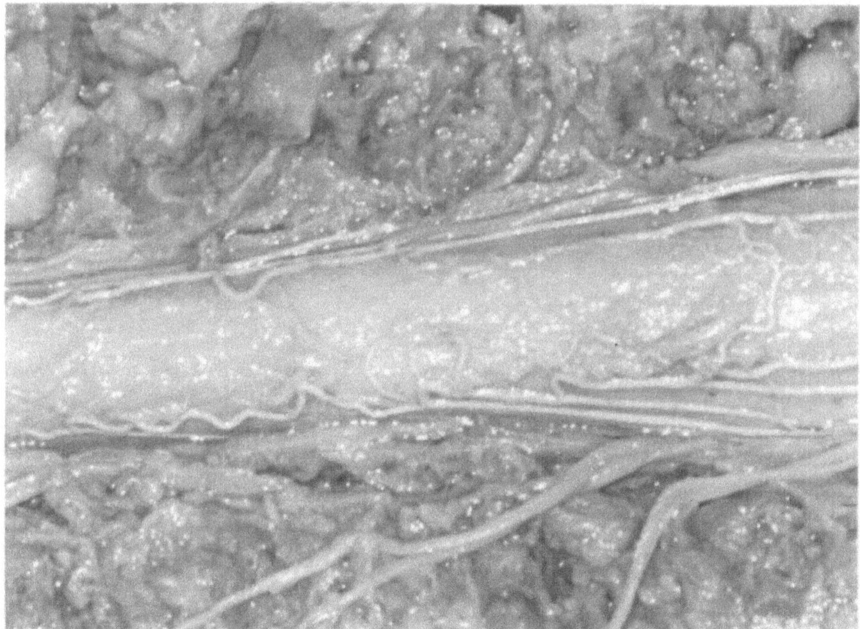

Fig. 43.   Cadaver. 3492. The postero-lateral arterial trunks at T.7–T.9 level with feeder
            arteries at T.7 & 8 right and T.8 level on the left side. The nerve rootlets are
            retracted and divided. (x16).

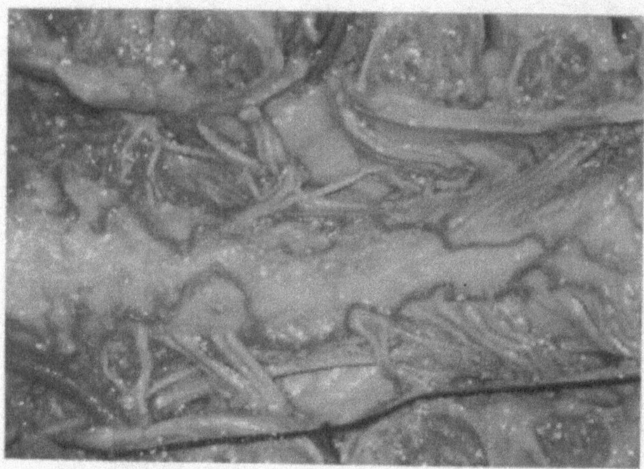

Fig. 44.   Cadaver 3210. The posterior aspect of the spinal cord at medulla oblongata
level, extending distally to C.5. The vertebral artery communicates with
the postero-lateral arterial trunks on left and right sides. The calibre of
the black silk thread is approximately 150 micro-millimeters. (x16)

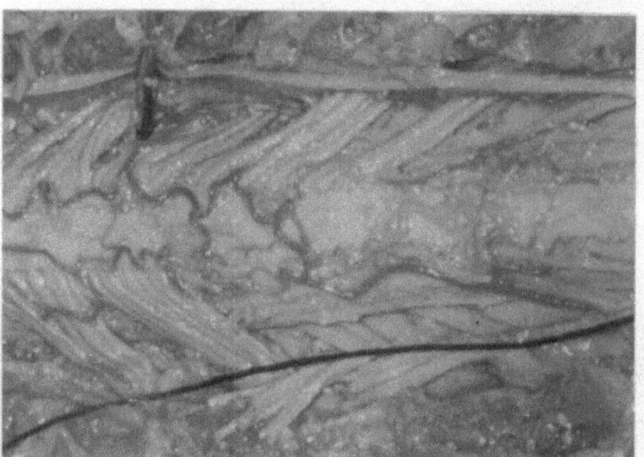

Fig. 45.   Cadaver 3210. The posterior arterial channels of the cord with the cord and
the nerve roots at C.6-T.2 level. The tortuous arterial channels communicate across the mid-line, and weave a course, now over now under the posterior nerve rootlets. The veins are unfilled and not evident. (x16).

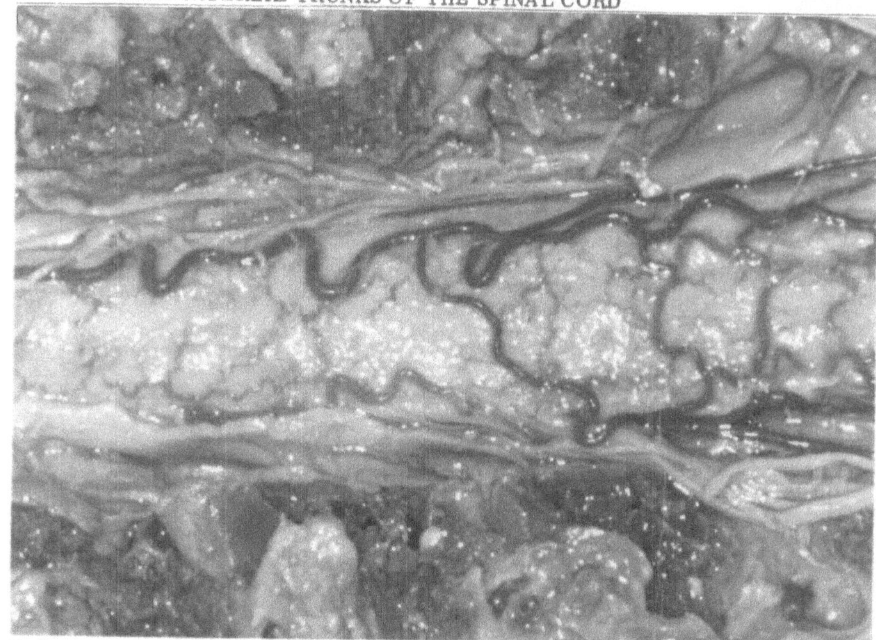

Fig. 46. Cadaver 3210. The posterior arterial trunks of the cord at T.9 to L.1 level.
The profuse communications between the two principal trunks are of arteriolar
proportion, approximately 20–32 micro-millimeters. Two large feeder vessels
occur on the right side at L.1 and L.3 levels, and on the left side at L.2 level.
The divided pedicles of the vertebrae, and two stumps of the segmental arteries
are clearly seen. (x16).

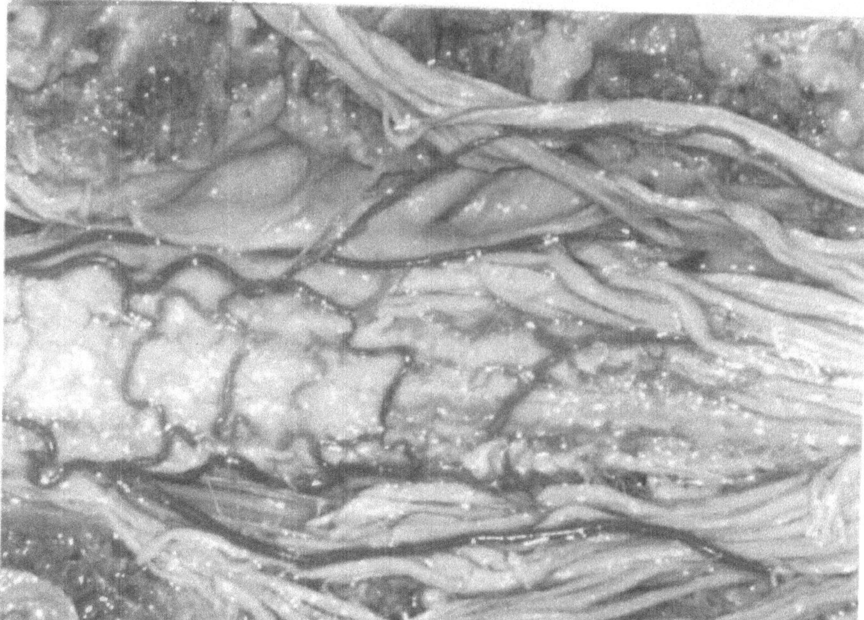

Fig. 47. The posterior aspect of the spinal cord and the conus medullaris with the rich
posterior arterial channels, feeders and transverse communicating vessels. At
the distal aspect of the cord, the postero-lateral channels are seen to be the
continuations in the opposite direction of the anterior median arterial trunk. (x16).

THE BLOOD SUPPLY OF THE SPINAL CORD

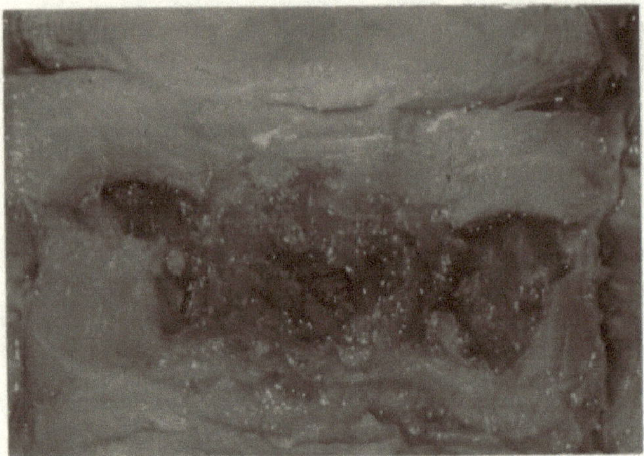

Fig. 48.   Cadaver 3184. Arterio-venous communications within the cancellous bone of the vertebral bodies are a normal phenomenon, and the injection material has shown the presence of large, blood-filled 'lakes'.

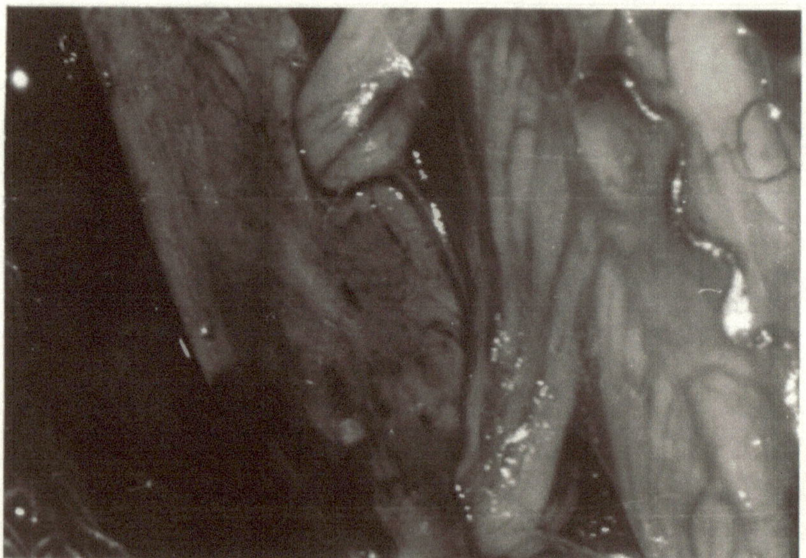

Fig. 49.   The appearances at an operation for decompression of the cervical roots. A thrombosed feeder vessel is seen accompanying the distal one of the 2 nerve roots, and the inference is that the radicular branch, for the supply of the nerve root, was also thrombosed. The patient suffered from cervical spondylosis. (Photo by courtesy of A. Rossouw). (x40)

DISCUSSION

Woollam and Millen (1958) observed: 'The principles on which the vascular architecture of the spinal cord is organised can be summarised in the form of a statement by Feeney and Watterson (1946). "There exists a very close relationship between the metabolic requirements of the nervous tissue and the final distribution of intraneural vessels in the adult, a relationship which functions in such a way as to provide the nervous system with a blood supply just adequate for its minimal needs." To put it in somewhat crude evolutionary terms, man has just as much nervous system as he can supply with oxygen and no more.'

There is yet another basic fact which the same authors stress: 'The poorest grey matter is indeed supplied with half as much again in capillary density as the richest white matter .... In any animal, the vascularity of both grey and white matter differs from situation to situation. The sensory nuclei have a richer supply than the motor nuclei; the ventral horns having, for example, fewer capillaries than the most poorly supplied sensory nuclei in the cord. In the white matter also there are very considerable differences from one area to another; the pyramidal tract, for example, being twice as profusely supplied with capillaries as the fasciculus cuneatus.'

While in the developing embryo there are to be found arterial vessels entering the spinal cord at every segmental level, the position alters so that when development is complete 'only a relatively few of these radicular arteries survive into adult life, from two to seventeen, with an average of eight.' (Woollam & Millen, 1958). In the present series, the variations in the number of anterior feeder vessels are also from 2-17, and the average number is 8, as reported also by Woollam and Millen, by Kadyi, (1889) and by Suh & Alexander, (1939).

Romanes (1965) is at variance in reporting that in a series of 22, '11 had four or fewer feeding vessles', while in the remaining 11 cadavers, there was only one with as many as ten. The factor responsible for this discrepancy is problematical, and does not appear to be related to age. In the series of Suh and Alexander, both adults and the newborn were included. Woollam resorted to the use of the guinea pig and rat for details of the early vascular pattern and to human cadavers for the adult. In another study, confined to the cervical cord, Turnbull et al. (1966), reporting on adults, having a mean age of 70 years, stated: 'the number of cervical anterior radicular arteries ranged from 1 to 6 ... (and) ... the number of posterior radicular arteries varied from 0 to 8 but three quarters of the specimens had either 2 or 3.' These figures are in close accord with the present series, in which the number of feeders ranges from 1 to 6 in respect of both the anterior and the posterior radicular arteries, in the cervical region of the cord.

THE REGIONAL DISTRIBUTION OF THE BLOOD SUPPLY OF THE CORD.

A glance at Plates I - VIII is sufficient to convince the reader that the greatest concentration of feeder arteries is at the cervical and the lumbar regions of the cord, where the concentration of grey matter is also greatest. Woollam & Millen, (1958) state: 'The reason for these variations remain to some extent a matter for speculation. Vascular density in the grey matter has been correlated with the number of synapses (Scharrer, 1944) and with oxidase content (Campbell, 1939) and the density of mitochondria in the neurons (Scharrer, 1945); all these factors indicating that the more metabolically active the area the better is its blood supply.'

Not only are the feeders largest and most numerous in the cervical and lumbar regions, but also the central perforating vessels which enter the median sulcus. These have been amply illustrated, (refer figs. 12-18), and their relative incidence in the different regions is: 'about 200 central branches in all, that is one to every 2mm. of spinal cord. In the human there are about 80 in the thoracic region, forty five in the cervical, 35 in the lumbar and 25 in the sacral region. Their *density* is, however, at its *lowest* in the thoracic region and at its greatest in the cervical and lumbar enlargements of the cord.' (Woollam & Millen).

THE DIRECTION OF FLOW IN THE ARTERIAL TRUNKS OF THE CORD.

Many observers have drawn conclusions from the experimental injection of blood vessels in the cadaver, and the variability of their conclusions bears witness to the unreliability of the technique. Fried et al. (1970), exposed the anterior aspect of the cervical spinal canal of the live rhesus monkey, and obtained a direct view of the anterior median arterial trunk of the cord in this area. Through a catheter inserted in the right brachial artery, they injected a dye and then took motion pictures at 48 frames per second of the coloured blood during its flow through the area. 'The flow of the dye in the anterior spinal artery was directed both cranially and caudally; a major component flowed rapidly up to C-2 level, while another flowed into the thoracic cord. The dye split either before or immediately after entering the anterior spinal artery, depending on the anatomical configuration of the feeding artery.' Woollam and Millen comment: 'It is extremely difficult to inject in human specimens and everything points to the view that the flow in the anterior spinal artery is directed from above and below towards the thoracic region.'

There is uncertainty about the direction of flow also at the proximal extremity of the cord where the anterior spinal arteries form communicating channels between the two vertebral arteries and the anterior median arterial trunk. In the series reported here, there is evidence that the flow may be in either a proximo-distal direction or the reverse, judging purely from the relative size of the respective vessels. In one instance, cadaver 3292 on Plate II, it would appear not unreasonable to assume that the flow is from one vertebral artery to the other. At the distal extremity of the cord, the picture is equally controversial, for while it is generally taken for granted that the direction of flow is from the distal extremity of the anterior median arterial trunk to the postero-lateral trunk on one or both sides via the posterior communicating arteries which are observed in the region of the conus medullaris, Romanes (1965) offers this valid comment: 'In the coccygeal part of the spinal cord there is a large communication between the anterior and posterior spinal arteries, and at this level the anterior spinal artery is suddenly reduced to a small vessel on the conus and filum terminale. The above communications, which are usually symmetrical but may be present on one side only, form the largest communication between the three longitudinal arteries at any level of the spinal cord. Between the entry of the great spinal artery (the artery of Adamkiewicz), and the origin of these communicating branches, the anterior spinal artery remains of relatively uniform calibre despite the number of branches arising from it, and this suggests the possibility that the communicating branches transmit blood to the anterior from the posterior spinal arteries, a possibility supported by the fact that large feeding vessels on the dorsal roots in the lumbar region send their major branches caudally. '

Arising from the investigations reported in this series, and supported by the presence of numerous extra-vertebral arterio-arterial anastomoses at all levels, it is suggested that the concept of a direction of flow should be replaced *by a concept of a complex and complicated arterial circle* in which the 3 longitudinal arterial trunks and their communications at all levels participate. This theory is no more than an extension of the principle of an arterial circle, such as the circle of Willis at the base of the brain. It implies a ready reversibility of flow and allows for an increased flow in any one direction, according to the momentary demand of a particular region. It is dependant for its continued effectiveness upon a constant arterial pressure within a complex system of channels which collectively form an 'arterial chamber', and it maintains a constant flow to the neural tissues via a multiplicity of outlets such as the perforating sulcal vessels. The small arteries on the surface of the cord, which pass between the anterior and posterior spinal vessels, may be regarded as additional outlets. In the event of a sudden excessive demand by one or another section, and also in the event of arterial obstruction, the arterio-arterial anastomoses, referred to by Lazorthes et al. (1971) as 'substitution pathways', and by Irvine et al. (1963) in regard to arterial communications between the external carotid and the vertebral arteries, could be instrumental in meeting sudden unusual demands. Chakravorty (1969), referred to the anastomoses between the spinal branches of the thyrocervical trunk and the vertebral artery, and concluded: 'It was apparent that either the vertebral or the ascending cervical can maintain the radicular supplies in the upper cervical region through these anastomoses if either source is blocked.'

The possibility of the arterio-arterial anastomoses acting to the disadvantage of the individual cannot be excluded, and as in the case of the 'subclavian arterial steal' referred to by Irvine et al. (1963), they could be instrumental in reversing the direction of the blood flow in the feeder (radicular) arteries. Pennybacker (1958) refers to both the acute and the sub-acute types of paraplegia, in which the findings at X-ray, the myelograms and the lumbar puncture are negative. He concludes: 'I suspect that in the majority it is a vascular lesion.'

THE ARTERIO- VENOUS ANASTOMOSES OF THE VERTEBRAL COLUMN (Fig. 48).

At the start of this project it became apparent that the injection material 'Revultex', which cannot penetrate to capillary or even pre-capillary level, was filling also the venous side of the circulation, and the possibility of arterio-venous anastomoses as a normal phenomenon in the spinal cord or the vertebral column was investigated by means of the dissections under the surgical microscope, i.e., by the process of macro- rather than micro-scopic dissection. Their presence has been recorded elsewhere, in the juxta-medullary renal glomeruli by Trueta and co-workers (1947), in the uterine endometrium by Schlegel (1944), and to the best of my knowledge also in the alveolar circulation of the lungs. In this series they were found only within the cancellous structure of the bones, both in the vertebral bodies and between the inner and outer diploic layers of the skull. They were not found within the neural tissues. In the vertebral bodies they were seen as large blood-filled lakes, which were supplied by nutrient arteries and drained by numerous veins which at all times appeared more numerous and larger than the arteries. (Fig. 48).

SOME PATHOLOGICAL ASPECTS OF THE BLOOD SUPPLY OF THE SPINAL CORD.

Impairment of the circulation of the spinal cord is of prime clinical importance. Romanes (1965) commented: 'It is obvious from the short period of absolute anoxaemia which the spinal cord can survive without permanent damage, that there is little possibility for the effective enlargement of a collateral circulation and that survival or death of spinal tissue following injury to the vascular supply must depend on the adequacy of the channels remaining intact. It is of some importance therefore, to determine which of the features of this blood supply are standard and which are liable to marked variation before attempting to predict the results of injury to different parts of this system.'

Trevor Hughes, (1965) groups the possible sites of arterial obstruction under seven headings, which include the vertebral arteries, the paired segmental arteries at all levels, the anterior and posterior feeder (radicular) arteries and all the small arteries arising from the anterior and the postero-lateral arterial trunks of the spinal cord. He includes also the veins of the cord, with this comment that 'the reserve of venous drainage (is so great) that venous obstruction rarely damages the spinal cord.' With this grouping and with the comment on the venous drainage, the writer is in agreement.

No thesis or dissertation on the clinical application of the blood supply of the spinal cord to the practice of surgery is complete without reference to the monumental work of the late Lionel Wolman, (1965) in respect of the nature of the vascular lesions in traumatic paraplegia. Wolman reported on the findings of 95 post-mortem examinations, and classified the lesions into early and late. In the former group there were intra-spinal haemorrhage, contusion, compression and thrombosis. In the late group, there were haemorrhage, haematomyelia, and arterial changes in the form of recanalisation of vessels. The latter phenomenon was seen in cases surviving one year or more. Wolman's conclusions in respect of traumatic haemorrhage were to the effect that subarachnoid and intra-spinal haemorrhages were the significant lesions, and that sub-dural and extra-dural haemorrhages were 'rare and never sufficiently severe to cause compression of the cord.'

The problem of cervical spondylosis and myelopathy as a result of arterial impairment in the canal of the vertebral artery has enjoyed much attention, and the classic work of Frykholm, (1951) has done much to promote understanding. In the matter of root pains or 'radiculitis', which are common accompaniments of the cervical syndrome, the explanation usually offered is of nerve root pressure due to foraminal narrowing by osteophytes. In a remarkable microphotograph taken during operation for laminectomy and decompression, and hitherto unpublished, Rossouw, (1972) has demonstrated thrombosis of a radicular vessel within the sub-dural space, and atresia of the accompanying nerve root which presents a withered appearance when compared with its healthy companion. (Fig. 49).

THE SIGNIFICANCE OF THE PAIRED SEGMENTAL ARTERIES OF THE SPINAL COLUMN.
In anterior surgical approaches to the vertebral column for conditions such as scoliosis, it is necessary to divide and ligate a varying number of the segmental arteries on the side of the approach. Anxiety on the part of the surgeon lest he precipitate a partial or total paraplegia is universally experienced. In a series of 127 operations in which the number of vessels ligated varied from 3 to 16, Dwyer, (1972) has reported no single instance of paraplegia due to cord ischaemia. In one instance, and at a follow-up operation, Dwyer ligated the 10th thoracic segmental artery on the other side also, again without ill effect. Hodgson, (1972) recalls 1 paraplegia in over 100 operations for spinal tuberculosis, which he attributes to ligation of segmental vessels. In a personal series of 29 operations, the author has recorded paraplegia in which a vascular factor could have been responsible, but could not be proved.

The artery of Adamkiewicz is a factor which is taken into consideration at operation, and reference to Plate IV cadaver 3247, in this series, offers a convincing reason: there are only two feeder arteries in this specimen, so that ligation of one of them could and probably would have had serious consequences. Unfortunately, there is no means of deducing the pattern of the spinal cord vascularisation in any individual patient, and there is only one manner in which it may be determined, namely, by means of selective angiography. This procedure is accordingly advised as a preliminary investigation in the type of case in which the circulation of the cord is likely to be compromised, either by the pathological condition present, or as a result of a surgical procedure. Keim & Hilal, (1971) of New York, have reported a series of 33 spinal angiographic investigations in scoliosis patients, without complications attributable to the procedure.

PARAPLEGIA & SCOLIOSIS

The threat of the development of paraplegia in the course of the management of scoliosis is always present, and is constantly in the mind of the spinal surgeon. It is a sinister threat, and a disastrous complication which may develop without known reason. A CRITICAL ZONE OF THE CORD is postulated.

THE CRITICAL ZONE OF THE SPINAL CORD.

Evidence brought forward in support of the postulate includes a number of factors referred to in the text above, factors which are to be taken into account also during the course of surgical procedures directed at the correction of major scoliosis deformity:

1.   LIGATION OF THE ARTERY OF ADAMKIEWICZ.   There has been no direct evidence to prove that ligation of this particular vessel, which is variable as to site and size, is critical. Reference to Plate IV, cadaver 3247, in which there are only two arterial feeder vessels, does however provide food for thought and should indicate the need for caution at least until the presence of other feeders in a particular instance has been demonstrated.

2.   THE SEGMENTAL ARTERIES OF THE VERTEBRAL COLUMN.   Ligation of numbers of these vessels, generally referred to as intercostal and lumbar arteries, has been reported in 3 series which total more than 250 operations: the over-all incidence of paraplegia was 3 from all causes, just over 1%.

3.   THE NARROW ZONE OF THE SPINAL CORD.   Dissections have revealed a narrow zone in the upper-mid-region of the thoracic spine of infants, (Refer Fig. 21), and accordingly the width of the canal in a series of cases, by means of radiological assessment has been calculated.   Fifty patients whose ages varied from 18 months to 68 years were included in the series, and the films were taken at standard distance with the patient standing erect. The inter-peduncular distance was measured over the entire thoracic and lumbar regions. A NARROW ZONE of the spinal canal was detected, involving either 4 or 5 vertebral segments from T.4 to T.8 in 50% of the series, and extending to T.3 or higher in 20% of instances, and to T.9 or lower in 30% of cases.

4.   THE DURAL MEMBRANE. In the infant, the vascularity and the thickness of the membrane were noteworthy features, (Figs. 8, 16, 20, 41, 42), in the absence of signs of inflammation or other pathological lesion. It was the impression of the writer that in the event of swelling of this membrane from whatever cause, encroachment upon the lumen of the canal would result at all levels, more particularly in the narrowest area.

Attention was also directed to the axillary pouches, (Fig. 20), the site of entry of the feeder arteries into the spinal canal in company with the nerve roots. In nearly every instance, the artery is enclosed in the radicular sheath during its passage through the axillary pouch; thickening of the axillary sheath , whether due to oedema, or to chronic fibrosis in association with osteo-arthritis, could be the cause of arterial constriction, more particularly in the narrow zone, for purely mechanical reasons.

5.   THE REGIONAL BLOOD SUPPLY OF THE SPINAL CORD. The relatively poor supply of the thoracic cord and the richer supply in the cervical and lumbar regions have been noted. When related to the presence of a narrow zone, then this factor assumes greater significance. The median arterial trunk is smaller and at the end of the supply route of blood from proximal and distal sources. The pressure of delivery of injection material is usually lower in this part of the artery in cadaveric specimens. The perforating, central sulcal vessels are fewer and smaller, and therefore more susceptible to increases in the normal intra-spinal pressure.

6.   THE ARTERIO-ARTERIAL ANASTOMOSES OF THE VERTEBRAL COLUMN. The presence of arterial circles at all levels has been noted, (Fig. 20, Figs. 22-27). The manner in which they could act to the advantage or the disadvantage of the spinal cord has been briefly referred to in the text.

7.   VENOUS OBSTRUCTION. The plexus of Batson surrounds the dural sac in a complex, complicated series of ill-defined channels which are joined together in a manner which resembles lacework. Trevor Hughes offers the opinion that the reserves of venous drainage are adequate to cope with the situation in all but the rarest instances. The matter is nevertheless controversial although it is not offered as a possible factor in spinal cord ischaemia in this presentation.

8.   CLINICAL AND POST-MORTEM EVIDENCE. In a recent unique series of cases reported by Dwyer, (1972) the onset of paraplegia has been recorded in 4 patients while undergoing treatment for scoliosis by means of the procedure known as halo-pelvic traction. The unique feature of these cases is the fact that the spinal cord is submitted to equal forces at all levels at one and the same time. It is reasonable to assume that in the event of embarrasment of the circulation of the spinal cord, such embarrassment would be effective at the vulnerable area, if indeed such an area is present. While it is too early to jump to conclusions, it is of interest to note that the post-mortem findings in 2 cases which proved fatal,

were of central necrosis of the spinal cord 'over about 4 or 5 segments, and the anterior spinal artery was still intact. The necrosis extended from D.5 to D.9 approximately, and the only recognizable anatomical structure practically was the anterior spinal artery ...'

The post-mortem findings in the only 2 cases records available to the writer, would seem to offer a degree of corroboration of the presence of a critical zone of the spinal cord, extending over 4 or 5 vertebral segments, centred upon T.6 vertebral segmental level.

SUMMARY AND CONCLUSIONS

The arterial blood supply of the spinal cord of the still-born human foetus at or near full term, and of the human neonate has been investigated with the aid of intra-arterial injections delivered via the femoral artery, and by means of micro-surgical dissections. The detailed findings in respect of the anterior vessels of 21 specimens and the posterior vessels of 9 specimens are presented. In 3 instances, both the anterior system and the posterior system of vessels of the same specimen are recorded, and the absence of any kind of formula or pattern relating one system to the other is noted.

The presence of a critical, narrow zone of the spine is postulated, and evidence is presented in support of the postulate.

The advantages of a method of study of the subject with the spinal cord 'in situ' are demonstrated in the findings, which relate to the source of the feeder arteries at all levels, and to the presence of multiple extra-vertebral arterio-arterial anastomoses. In addition, the intimate relationship between the vessels of the cord and those of surrounding structures is demonstrated.

The vertebral artery has been shown to be the dominant vessel in the supply of feeder arteries of the cord in the neck. Forty-nine of a total of 62 cervical cord feeders in the series were branches of the vertebral artery in the course of its passage up the transverse foramina.

The direction of flow of the circulation of the cord has been discussed and a tentative explanation in which the principle of a pressure chamber with multiple supply sources and multiple outlet points is postulated.

The role of the anterior spinal branches of the vertebral artery at the cranial end of the cord, and of the posterior communicating arteries which connect the anterior to the postero-lateral arterial trunks in the region of the conus medullaris, has been discussed in the light of the possible reversibility of the blood flow in these channels.

At the most distal level, the lateral sacral artery has been shown to supply anterior feeder arteries of moderate size only in 33% of the specimens examined.

The pattern of the blood vessels of the human spinal cord at birth is described in 27 cadavers of full-term foetuses and of neonates. An outstanding feature throughout has been the constancy of the principle and the variability of the pattern – the richest supply being found in the regions of the greatest demand, viz. the cervical and the lumbar enlargements. Individual patterns of supply cannot be deduced from a study of the average pattern.

THE BLOOD SUPPLY OF THE SPINAL CORD

<u>REFERENCES</u>

ADAMKIEWICZ, A.A. (1881):	Ueber die mikrokopischen Gefässe des menschlichen Rückenmarkes. Trans. 7th Session, Int. Med. Congr. Vol. I, pp. 155-157.
IBID, (1881):	S.B. Akad. Wiss Wien (Math.-nat K.L.) 84,469.
IBID, (1882):	Die Blutgefässe des menschlichen Rückenmarkes: II. Die Gefässe der Rückenmarksoberfläche, Situngsb. d.k. Akad. d. Wissensch., Math.-naturw. C1. 85: 101-130.
BOLTON, B. (1939):	"The Blood Supply of the Human Spinal Cord". Journ. Neurol. Psychiat. N.S. 1-2, 137-148.
CAMPBELL, A.C.P. (1939):	Arch Neurol. Psychiat. 41, 223.
CRAIGIE, E. (1955):	In: Biochem of the Developing Nervous System. Edited by H. Waelsh. New York. page 28.
CHAKRAVORTY, B.G. (1969):	The Arterial Supply of the Cervical Cord and its relation to Cervical Spondylosis in Myelopathy. Annals Roy. Coll. Surg. Eng., 45, 232-251.
DI CHIRO, G., FRIED, L.C. & DOPPMAN, J.L. (1970):	"Experimental Spinal Cord Angiography". Br. J. Radiol. 43, 19-30.
DOMMISSE, G.F. (1972):	"Some factors in the management of Fractures & Fracture-Dislocations of the Spine at Lumbo-dorsal level. The Significance of the Blood Supply of the Spine." Reconstruction Surgery & Traumatology. Vol. 13 (in Press).
DWYER, A.F. (1972):	Personal Communication.
FEENEY, J.F., AND WATTERSON, R.L. (1946):	Journ. Morph., 78, 231.
FRIED,L.C., DOPPMAN, J.L. AND DI CHIRO, G. (1970):	"Direction of Blood Flow in the primate cervical spinal cord." J. Neurosurg. 33, 325-330.
FRYKHOLM, R.:	Lower Cervical Vertebrae and Inter-vertebral Discs. Surgical Anatomy & Pathology. Acta Chir. Scand. 101: 345-359.
HODGSON, A.R., (1972):	Personal communication.
HOLDSWORTH,F.W. AND HARDY, A. (1953):	"Early Treatment of Paraplegia from Fractures of the Thoraco-Lumbar Spine." Journal of Bone and Joint Surg. 35B. 540.

HUTCHINSON, E.C. &
YATES, P.O. (1956):
"The Cervical Portion of the Vertebral Artery.
A clinico-path. study. Brain, 79, 319-331.

IRVINE, W.T., LUCK, R.J.,
SUTTON, D. AND D. WALPITA, P.R.
(1963):
Intrathoracic Occlusion of Great Vessels Causing Cerebrovascular Insufficiency. Lancet,
7292, Vol. 1, 117-1181.

KADYI, H. (1889):
Ueber die Blutgefässe des menschlichen
Rückenmarkes; nach einer im XV. Bande der
Denkschriften der math.-naturw. Classe der
Akademie der Wissenschaften in Krakau
erschienenen Monographie, aus dem Polnischen
übersetzt vom Verfasser, Lemberg, Poland,
Gubrynowicz & Schmidt.

KEIM, H.A., AND
HILAL, S.K. (1971):
Spinal Angiography in Scoliosis Patients.
Journal of Bone & Joint Surg., 53-A, 5, 904.

LAZORTHES. G., GOUAZE, A.,
ZADEH, J.O., SANTINI, J.J.,
LAZORTHES, Y., & BURDIN, P. (1971):
Arterial vascularization of the spinal cord.
Recent studies of the anastomotic substitution
pathways. J. Neurosurg. 35, 253-262.

PENNYBACKER, J., (1958):
In: Discussion on Vascular Disease of the
Spinal Cord. Proc. Royal Soc. Med. 51, 547.

ROMANES, G.J., (1965):
"The Arterial Blood Supply of the Human Spinal
Cord". Paraplegia. 2. 4. 199-207.

ROSSOUW, A., (1972):
Personal Communication.

SCHARRER, E., (1944):
Quart. Rev. Biol., 19, 308.

IBID., (1945):
J. Comp. Neurol., 83, 237.

SCHLEGEL, J.U., (1945/46):
Arteriovenous Anastomoses In The Endometrium In Man. Acta Anat. 1, 284-325.

STREETER, G.L. (1918):
"The Developmental Alterations in the Vascular
System of the Brain of the Human Embryo."
Carnegie Inst. Washington, Contributions to
Embryology. 8.

SUH, T.H. &
ALEXANDER, L. (1939):
Vascular System of the Human Spinal Cord.
Arch. Neurol. Psychiat. 41, 659.

TREVOR HUGHES, J. (1965):
The Pathology of Vascular Disorders of the
Spinal Cord. ,PARAPLEGIA, 2,4, 207-213.

TRUETA, J., BARCLAY, A.E.,
DANIEL, P.M., FRANKLIN, K.J. &
PRICHARD, M.M.L., (1947):
Studies of the Renal Circulation. London &
Oxford, A.R. Mowbray & Co. Ltd.
Blackwell Scientific Publications.

TURNBULL, I.M., BRIEG, A.
& HASSLER, O.:
Blood Supply of Cervical Spinal Cord in Man.
Journ. of Neurosurgery, 24: 1966. pp. 951-965.

WOLMAN, LIONEL (1965):   The Disturbance of Circulation in Traumatic Paraplegia in Acute and Late Stages: A Pathological Study. PARAPLEGIA, 2,4, 213-226.

WOOLLAM, D.H.M. & MILLEN, J.W. (1958):   In: Discussion on Vascular Diseases of the Spinal Cord. Proc. Roy. Soc. Med. 51, 540.